PHYSICIANS AND HOSPITALS:

EASING ADVERSARY RELATIONSHIPS

RICHARD E. THOMPSON, M.D.

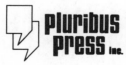

pluribus press inc.

Library of Congress Catalog Card Number:
84-60124

International Standard Book Number:
0-931028-49-3

Pluribus Press, Inc., Division of Teach 'em, Inc.
160 East Illinois Street
Chicago, Illinois 60611

Printed in the United States of America

Physicians and Hospitals: Easing Adversary Relationships

Contents

Part I: The First Key: Understanding What We Know About Doctors and Hospitals

Part II: The Second Key: Really Believing That It's Not "Business As Usual" for Hospital Executives or Practitioners

Part III: The Third Key: We Know the Similarities Between Hospitals and Commercial Industry; It's Time to Talk About the Differences

Part IV: The Fourth Key: Facing Up to Reality

Part V: The Fifth Key: New Practical Approaches

Preface

The history of physician/hospital executive/board relations is stormy at best. Relations that have improved in recent years are once again threatened because hospitals and practitioners find themselves at mutual peril. Mistakes made by hospital managers can impact adversely on practitioners' interests in economic, legal, and altruistic patient-care sense. Errors made by practitioners who respond inappropriately to the panic of economic pressures could devastate a hospital. Both hospitals and practitioners find themselves suddenly forced to operate in a buyer's market. Some pessimistic observers predict that the hospital management/hospital staff alliance will not survive this, its sternest test. Some predict that the outcome will be disastrous because medical staff members and hospital managers will engage in locking antlers in a bloody death struggle, rather than working together to sort out what is big business about modern health care and what is compassionate caring.

Others (including this author) believe something quite different.

> These new times provide the opportunity to shake off mistaken assumptions of a quarter century of misdirected initiatives, superficiality and artificiality in selecting goals

> and methods for achieving quality
> patient care at reasonable cost and
> with reasonable accessibility.

It won't be easy. The discussions in this book are challenging and the specific practical suggestions with which this book concludes are not for the timid.

But then, being either a healthcare executive concerned with hospital care as big business, or being a practitioner accepting responsibility for the health and safety of the human individual within current constrained economic times, is not a role for the timid.

Business and Patient Care

The success of the American healthcare industry in its broadest sense and the hopes and fears of specific individuals requiring healthcare services, especially of complex technologic nature, as well as the future of both administrators and practitioners employed in the healthcare field have never before been so inextricably intertwined.

> At this juncture in the history of the
> American healthcare scene, those
> with business backgrounds who
> insist on viewing healthcare as big
> business *only* will fail in one way. On
> the other hand, practitioners who
> believe their independent judgments

> and self-reliance are sufficient in a complicated technological healthcare world will fail in another way.

We've always known that we'd have to get it together. There is no need for a fatalistic assumption that it is too late.

If this book turns just a few heads away from counter productive turf-guarding and adversary position taking toward effective, cooperative problem solving, then its objective will be met.

Move Over Machiavelli

Hospitals are experiencing the consequences of the adversary, manipulative environment of the 1970s. These consequences are reflected in current buzzwords: "economic survival," "turf guarding," "image problem," "liability," etc.

Trends in other industries suggest the discovery (rediscovery, actually) of a more open, communicative management approach. In hospitals, as well as in other industries, one expected reward is increased productivity. But in hospitals, a politically sensitive industry, an additional reward is a much-needed base of support among employees, medical staff members, the press, politicians, and local business leaders. Indeed, the ability to replace suspicion and frustration with understanding and trust may be the secret weapon of the truly successful "preferred provider" of the 1980s and 1990s.

It's tempting to include here a list of the numerous interfaces presented by the multi-faceted hospital organization (administration and nursing, board and the community it represents, personnel ["human resources" and hospital employees], hospitals in the business community, nurses and the medical staff, etc.), but the greater need seems to be for specific, detailed suggestions focusing on *methods* by which executives/managers and physicians/medical staff can overcome their conditioned, adversary response to each other. More than a language barrier is involved.

Richard E. Thompson, M.D.

Introduction

This Book Tells:

- How hospital management and medical staff can work together to reconcile the realities of mandated DRG reimbursement on one hand, with, "The government's not going to tell me how to practice medicine," on the other.

- How doctors view the "incident reporting" mechanism, which is implemented by the nursing department, as a new spy system imposed by administration. Yet, knowledge about "incidents" is important for many reasons. What should be done?

- How to handle confrontations. *Example:* Hospital management has responded to economic times by opening an ambulatory-care satellite in a shopping center near the hospital. The medical staff calls this the administrator's pet "Doctor-in-the-box" project, claims that the medical staff had no input into the decision, and is calling for the board to fire the administrator because he does not "deal from a straight deck" with the medical staff. Could this confrontation have been avoided? How?

- How to resolve delicate medical staff issues. *Example:* Hospital counsel advises the medical staff executive committee that if they do not process the application from the podiatrist, legal jeopardy may result. The key physician leader's position is, "We don't think we ought to just roll over for these guys and let them do anything they want to in the hospital." The executive committee even wonders if they can trust the hospital's legal counsel and wonders if the medical staff should have its own legal counsel. How can this situation be resolved?

• What to do with the truculent physician. *Example:* One "key physician leader" is persistently negative and disruptive. He calls "rump group" meetings of the medical staff at his house and frequently writes fiery letters to individual hospital board members whom he has known for years. When asked to use organized medical staff channels, including the Joint Conference Committee, he replies, "My kind of politics is to take my patients to another hospital, not to come to board meetings." What, if anything, can be done?

If, in your hospital, management and the medical staff are dealing with any issue that is presently stalemated and both "sides" feel that they have "tried everything," this book may suggest a way to go back to square 1, take a different run at the problem, and discover a solution.

PART I
The First Key:
Understanding What We Know
About Hospitals and Doctors

CHAPTER 1

Root cause of conflict: a lack of understanding no one wants to admit

Physicians, in years of training and practice, may learn little about the hospital on which they so greatly depend.

A few years ago, while cleaning out the basement, I stumbled across the vocations paper I wrote years ago as a senior in high school. As I read what I had written at age 18, I was mortified and embarrassed. But the next feeling to sweep over me was a realization that I had discovered, on those dusty pages, a crystal-clear insight about the level of the average physician's understanding of the hospital as an organization.

"My choice is between the 3 M's . . . Music, Medicine, and the Ministry," I wrote. I went on to say that I was currently leaning toward the field of medicine. "In terms of what kind of doctor I want to be," I continued glibly (sans any kind of research), "the way I understand it, I have two choices: I can either go to medical school, get a license to practice, set up an office, and start treating patients. Or, I can get the M.D. degree, then go to work at the hospital as an intern and work my way up to superintendent."

The superficial humor of that incident is apparent, but the deeper tragedy may not be. The tragedy is that during four years of medical school, three years of residency, and eight years of private practice, my understanding of the hospital really did not grow far beyond that adolescent misconception.

It has now occurred to me that perhaps lay board members, and even trained managers and executives, may not really understand the hospital. Today, a high school senior preparing to be a hospital administrator or president might write a vocational paper stating that:

- hospitals are *big business* and must be run like big business

- hospitals must be tightly structured like any other business corporation to accomplish this goal

- as with any good business corporation, total control must reside with the president

- the major drawback to entering hospital administration is a huge obstacle to this businesslike approach—the medical staff. The medical staff, the student might write, is the wart on this perfect corporate structure and is to be dealt with very carefully and as little as possible.

> Hospital managers and physicians can never work together productively until both groups recognize that today's hospital is, in reality, more complex than either group's sometimes short-sighted, simplistic, obsolete perception.[1]

[1] Read "Is the Hospital Beyond Our Understanding?," by Basil Mott, *Trustee*, pp. 21—25. April 1981.

CHAPTER 2

Seven little-acknowledged facts

Let's face it. The hospital industry is struggling and so is the medical profession. Struggling with DRG reimbursement, competitive strategies and the new vanguard of industrial coalitions. Struggling with legal problems like malpractice, restructuring, and the definition of death. Struggling with an image problem, hoping they don't make "60 Minutes."

Traditional efforts, such as jumping on one bandwagon after another and being aggressive with legal actions, hasn't stopped the tailspin. In fact, some of the things hospitals and doctors have done make the problems worse instead of better.

The President's Commission on Malpractice concluded that people believe the informed consent mechanism is designed to protect hospitals and doctors from lawsuits, rather than to provide information to the patient. That's true, of course. And if you wonder why the DRG-payment system was imposed on hospitals, imagine a situation in which industry, government, and consumers are worried about healthcare costs, yet see hospitals flaunt their avowed goal of being profit-making conglomerates.

The secret weapon of the truly preferred provider of the 1980s and 1990s is to find truly innovative approaches to old and new problems. To do that, hospital executives/managers and medical staff members alike will have to face up to seven seldom-mentioned facts:

1. Most physicians do not understand the hospital as an organization and the nature of pressures upon it. Neither do they understand the medical staff as an organization. There is little distinction on the part of most doctors between what the *medical staff organization* does and what an individual physician does.

    A part of this problem is that most members of the organized medical staff do not relate to the medical staff bylaws as a useful instrument, or even know what provisions the medical staff bylaws contain.

2. In hospitals, people with business and management backgrounds are taking approaches to physicians that make sense to people with business and management backgrounds. *Example:* "How can we get the doctor to come to the risk management committee meeting and participate in the risk management program?" To a physician, risk is another term for day-to-day, individual clinical decision making. Physicians are constantly at risk because of the degree of uncertainty with which they must live when making clinical decisions. To make "risk" sound like a matter of a "committee meeting" or a "program" does not ring true to the physician.

    When hospital management does consider the physician, it may be in such terms as "how to involve a physician as a member of the hospital management team." Many hospitals are now deciding whether they need the services of a medical director or vice president of professional affairs, but that's not the way to frame the *basic* question. The basic question is, "How can hospital management truly involve the medical staff in hospital affairs, and make sure that 'grass roots' medical staff members *know* that they are involved?"

3. Business and management people tend to run on one of only two speed settings: Fast run and sprint.

4. Physicians tend to accept change at one of only two speed settings: Slowly and not at all.

5. Time spent developing understanding (bridging the gap between three and four) has not traditionally been considered productive time.

6. Most people tend to fix the blame, not the problem. We should try to recognize that no one is to blame for the basic pressure on us all—change—and to rediscover cooperative problem solving as an amazingly effective answer to, "How do you spell relief?" in conflict situations.

7. Some hospital administrators act as if they can do without doctors. They're the administrators who are always updating their resumés. Conversely, some doctors seem to think they can do without trained hospital executives/managers. They see a weak board as a medical staff advantage. They're the doctors who are always finding new ways to make themselves vulnerable through actions they consider protective.

> As the economic, legal, image, and ethical pressures on hospital executives and practitioners become more complex, no one can hope to win with only half a team.

CHAPTER 3

The players: evolution
of the relationship

The average medical man is an educated gentleman, a delightful companion, a man of parts, and many such are our best friends; but doctors, when associated in corporate matters, are oftentimes too self-seeking. With an eye out for their profession, they are inclined to be aggressive, and naturally, under such conditions are not a gracious, peaceful, easily cooperative body of men. This professional enthusiasm is apt to obscure an all-around view of hospital government.

"Observations on Hospital Organization"
George H.M. Rowe, M.D.
Association of Hospital Superintendents
1902

Now the physician, unless he's a real great guy, spends his day vaulting fences. He orders new equipment, fires nurses, reduces bills, and writes all sorts of libelous remarks in the medical records—if he writes at all. But this type of physician is pretty much a vanishing breed. He's been worn down, or perhaps matured, or maybe both. . . .

The chief executive officer is the least likely to jump his fence—at least twice. He gets fired after the first time

> . . . he may be the chief executive officer, but he's no dictator. He has learned that to be successful he must be not only right, but right at the right time, in the right manner, and with the right people. That complicates administration, but that's the way things are.
>
> *Hospitals Are Us*
> Robert R. Cadmus, M.D.
> Teach 'Em, Inc., 1979

Negative Perceptions: A Loss of Respect Somewhere Along the Way

Disagreements between professional "doers" and company management are nothing new. Such disagreements usually result in negative perceptions of the other individual or group. "Management is not dealing from a straight deck." "Management doesn't care about progress or people—only about profits." So say the professionals. "Those spoiled tinkerers think we have all the money in the world for them to try out every fly-by-night idea." So says management.

This scenario is common—a familiar old movie storyline. The eager young innovator (usually Gary Cooper or Jimmy Stewart) fights against odds for the financial backing of a large company. In the movie, of course, the innovations always work, and the innovator gets respect, the president's daughter, and the number two spot in the company.

In real life it doesn't always work that way. The battles over space, equipment, and personnel can lead to bitter, deep-rooted lack of respect between technical professionals and management professionals. Compromise, not victory, may turn out to be the real-world solution.

Hospitals Are No Exception

In a telephone poll, fifty doctors were asked to say what they thought of hospital administrators, and fifty hospital administrators were asked to describe physicians ("Cooperation or conflict: Physicians vs. administrators" *Hospitals*, July 16, 1979). Here's a sampling of the results.

Hospital administrators said that physicians were:

- egotistical bumblers, who resented and envied the better organizational skills of administrators

- tinkerers who want the most expensive, latest, technological gadgetry to play with

- above-average people in some ways, yet immature in getting along with others

- independent thinkers who unrealistically deny the reality that when they come to the hospital they are part of an organization

- confused about their responsibilities and authority in the hospital

- not adept at interpersonal relations

- fundamentally unequipped to deal with non-medical matters

Physicians said that hospital administrators/executives were:

- aloof, insecure bureaucrats

- concerned more with cost accounting than with patient care

- trying to deal with things that should be dealt with by the medical staff. *Example:* Handling the problem of an alcoholic physician

- making decisions (where to cut costs, reduce nursing staff, or assign available space) without asking the medical staff for advice and input

- confused about their authority over and responsibility to the medical staff

- announcing meetings for the purpose of getting the doctors' opinions, but turning the meetings into lectures from the administration

- always at bat for the board, but never for the doctors

Incidentally, there was a common thread in these interviews. Physicians and administrators alike felt that . . .

> The basic problem is lack of effective communication, both in terms of effective organizational communication mechanisms and individual communication with each other.

CHAPTER 4

We've come a long
way . . . or have we?

In the good old days, a hospital represented a tranquil (usually) company of angels. In those days, the hospital was trusted and respected as a professional service institution, usually founded and nurtured by either church groups or local philanthropists.

In those days, the picture of hospital organization was pretty simple (see Figure 4-1). The patient sought attention from the physician who then brought the patient, if need be, to a workshop, the hospital. There, the physician was the unquestioned captain of the ship or, at worst, one of the three legs of a stool. (We continue to seek just the right analogy to fit the reality of a hospital practice when no exact analogy exists.) At the hospital, eagerly and enthusiastically awaiting the orders of the captain of the ship, were at least the following groups:

Board of Trustees—They presided over the business side of things—buildings, equipment purchasing, remodeling the laundry—that sort of thing. At the end of the year, they reached into their own pockets to make up any funds necessary to assure that this hospital—their community's pride—would break even or be in the black. They would never presume, of course, to question or attempt to second guess any decisions made by members of the medical staff.

Figure 4-1

TRADITIONAL BUT OBSOLETE VIEW OF THE HOSPITAL

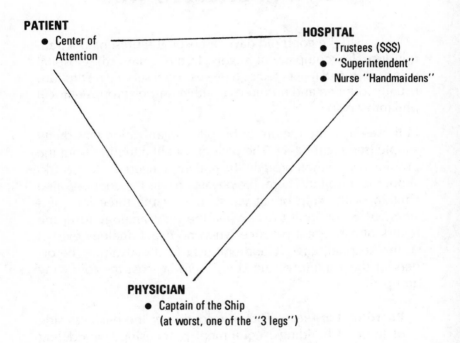

PATIENT
- Center of
  Attention

HOSPITAL
- Trustees ($$$)
- "Superintendent"
- Nurse "Handmaidens"

PHYSICIAN
- Captain of the Ship
  (at worst, one of the "3 legs")

Superintendent—Hospital board members have businesses of their own to run, and physicians make their rounds and then leave the hospital to go to the office, but somebody has to stay and administer daily affairs for the medical staff and board. This lucky person was the superintendent, or administrator (never the president).

Nursing Staff—The needs of the hospitalized patient were primarily met by these, the true angels of the company, who served as the physicians' handmaidens and stood respectfully when he came onto the ward to make daily rounds.

Various Hospital Personnel (Medical Records, Dietary, Housekeeping, etc.)—These individuals worked under the supervision of the superintendent. Yet, if they should inadvertently interfere with or anger a physician, the physician might threaten to fire them, on the spot. Very confusing.

In this "ideal" hospital, few restrictions were applied. Services to patients certainly were not restricted. The rule of thumb was "whatever it takes, and as often as needed," whether the statement related to days in the hospital, administration of drugs, oxygen, or blood, nursing care, or diagnostic or surgical procedures.

The hospital itself was not restricted. It (thanks to its founders and trustees) paid its own way. And, after all, who would want to restrict this trusted, respected, professional service institution?

Finally, were the physicians restricted? You've got to be kidding!

In a movie titled *Ride the Pale White Horse*, Anthony Quinn plays the prefect of police in a small town in the early 1900s. At one point in the film, he approaches the chief nurse of the local hospital. "The smuggler that has been hiding in the mountains has been wounded in the leg by my men," he informs her. "He surely will seek attention in this hospital. Until he is captured, we must encircle the hospital with police and not let anyone in or out."

In amazement, the chief nurse replies, "*Surely* you don't intend to restrict the movement of the *physicians*!"

Immediately the police captain responds, "Oh, of course, the *doctors* will be allowed to come and go as they please."

A basic problem for hospital managers and medical staff members alike is that physicians, traditionally accustomed to being the unquestioned captain of the ship, have to mesh with a complex healthcare team, and be subject to reasonable policies and rules just like everybody else.

> The only thing worse than doctors who don't understand that they're no longer the unquestioned captain of the ship are deluded hospital executives who think they're now king of the hill.

> While some individuals seem honestly to believe that the description of a hospital as unrestricted and unaccountable is still accurate, the date on this model is about 1776 to the 1950s.

A Shake Up On Cloud 9

Well, indeed, why couldn't the Company of Angels continue unrestricted?

The answer is medical technology—the industrial revolution in medical care—won't let it. The old hospital model fit when a patient with a heart attack was admitted, provided the best in supportive care along with specifically indicated drugs, and often even accorded the privacy and quiet of a "private room."

But the old model of a hospital does not fit the coronary care unit patient requiring an expert team to observe monitors, insert pacemakers, and replace obstructed natural coronary arteries with artificial, new ones.

> We often forget that the basic beginning point of the need for change in hospitals is amazing technical capability.

As these new capabilities evolved, the rule of thumb was, "Whatever it takes and as often as possible, for everybody." The reaction to this rule was enthusiastic and supportive. Therefore, by the early 1970s we had:

- Hill Burton funds to build more hospitals

- more medical schools to turn out increased numbers of physicians to perform these modern miracles

- area health education centers and regional medical programs to extend these miracles throughout the land

- programs to teach, train, orient, register, license, and certify a new army of physician extenders to provide the overworked and exhausted physicians with the capability of meeting the needs of more and more patients simultaneously. (Marcus Welby is the only doctor in the world who has only one patient at a time.)

> Hospital managers and physicians should constantly remind themselves and each other that many individuals with whom they work began their careers during this period of time. "Whatever it takes" was comfortable for physicians, and the goal of expansion was right in line with the teachings of business management. No wonder we're all having trouble adjusting to "containment" incentives.

A Troubling New Question: Who Pays?

During those glory years of health care, some wise heads were shaking and some experienced voices were asking, "Isn't paying for all this going to be somewhat of a problem?"

Of course the response was, "Not to worry! This is America. Money is no problem." The answer to "Who pays?" was, for some, *health insurance*. For others, the answer to "Who pays?" was *the government*.

The Company of Angels Adds Some Angels

Of course, the new angels such as the government and insurance companies were glad to provide funds *as long as* they were assured that the funds were used in good faith and trust. They began to insist on being involved in or, at the very least, having assurance of responsible decision making at the hospital. This included:

- clinical decisions made by the members of the medical staff
- management and policy decisions made by hospital managers and board members

Meanwhile, the patient in this new healthcare world took on several additional roles . . . taxpayer, voter, consumer.

> No longer the vine-covered, publicly trusted and respected, pay-your-own-way institution, hospitals saw the need to respond to new external influences by rearranging their internal organizational structure and function.

The Company of Angels Incorporates

Before the captains of the ships had time to understand why it was necessary, they found themselves replaced at the helm by the former superintendents, who now insisted on being called presidents. Before board members had a chance to understand it was happening, they were rudely dislodged from the role of revered senior community member and philanthropist and became directors who were expected to run the company in a hard-nosed way, following the lead of the new president.

In a development perhaps proving injurious in the long run, hospitals began to pursue the traditional goals of commercial big business: growth, profit, and eliminating the competition. Financial, accounting, legal, planning, and marketing services became the central hub of the hospital. The quiet corridors of these offices were carpeted, and those who inhabited them seldom stepped into the real world of clinical decision and daily practice. After all, too many financial, legal, accounting, price structuring, and data processing matters needed attention. There were committee meetings to staff, consultants to entertain. One did not have time for that *and* for being concerned with what went on between individual practitioner and individual patient.

The Effect on the Medical Staff

Without full explanations as to why (time spent developing understanding was not considered productive time), the medical staff suddenly discovered:

- New medical staff members were no longer elected by popular vote of the entire medical staff. Rather, applicants to the staff were recommended to the *board* for appointment. And the board's decision was *final*.

- The security of lifelong medical staff appointment had disappeared. One had to be *re*appointed every year or two.

- The superintendent seemed to hold too much power.

- The hospital seemed top-heavy on the management side.

- The nurses' relationship with management was closer than before, and, perhaps, was becoming even closer than the nurse-physician relationship.

- The once-proud captain of the ship was expected to scrub the decks for the president if requested.

- Trustees believed they ran the place.

- Medical staff bylaws were being hauled out, dusted off, and revised to include *obligations* of medical staff members, as well as privileges—unheard of.

- Most amazing of all—concerns of the medical staff regarding patient-care needs seemed to get little attention as hospital managers pursued their more lofty business goals.

- Physicians were expected to use their clinical expertise to review and pass judgment on each other's clinical practices.

The internal result of this upheaval was *not* an increasingly trusting relationship between physicians and hospital managers.

PART II:
The Second Key:
Really Believing That It's Not "Business as Usual" for Hospital Executives *or* Practitioners

CHAPTER 5

Bring back
the good old days

Wanted: Experienced hospital trustee to serve as member of the governing body of a non-profit, medium-sized hospital with full range of services, fiscally sound, and fully accredited. *Compensation Zero. Responsibility unlimited.* Must be committed to dealing with an extravagant range of problems in an over-regulated industry.

Wall Street Journal
Reported in *Trustee*, March, 1983

When it comes to quality and competition, the bottom line may best be characterized by noting the message that doctors in hospitals have received for at least a decade: "If you want things to stay at all the same, you must accept some change." Because of pressures of competition and cost cutting, this same advice now also applies to hospital executives and governing board members.

Richard E. Thompson, M.D.
"The Pendulum Swings"
Hospitals, June 16, 1983

Remember in the 1970s when we got PSRO, HSAs, required CME, JCAH's "audit" requirements, and the malpractice crisis? Remember how we longed for the good old days. Now we find those *were* the good old days. In one sense, the pressures on doctors and hospitals are the same in the 1980s as they were in the 1970s:

1. government

2. law

3. Joint Commission

4. money

5. medical staff

6. future

7. people

8. image

The difference—manifestations of those pressures have changed from a soft-shoe routine to a game of hardball.

The Government

One answer to the question, "What are 'TEFRA' and 'DRGs'?" is that they are the answer to the old 1970's question, "What could possibly be worse than PSRO?"

The Law

Traditional legal issues still exist: malpractice suits, corporate organization of a hospital, the definition of death. But new economic times bring new legal pressures. What is cooperation, and what is restraint of trade? What should be the status at the hospital of independent practitioners other than physicians and dentists?

Joint Commission on Accreditation of Hospitals

New standards and new, more functional survey procedures are making the Joint Commission certificate of much greater value. But the price is replacing the illusion of quality assurance (contrived studies, stacks of essay-type minutes, and little actual impact) with a genuine hospital-wide accountability system (objective information shared and dealt with by responsible individuals).

Money

There is no time in life for anyone when money is *not* an issue. In the healthcare field, the money pressures take the form of competition and new restrictive payment mechanisms.

Medical Staff

The medical staff is an issue to physicians, as in "too many committee meetings" and the question of "adequate medical staff input."

And the medical staff continues to be an issue to hospital executives, especially those from industrial backgrounds, as they try to solve the problem of how to bring the medical staff under their complete control.

Future

You can't just be a hospital anymore; you have to work at deciding what kind of hospital you want to be. A tragedy of recent times is exemplified by the chief executive officer who, in giving a talk to other chief executive officers on the topic of long-range planning, said, "When we encountered that problem we turned to the community, perhaps in desperation." Do hospitals turn to their communities for guidance in long-range planning only in desperation?

People

Communities of real people—patients and family members, taxpayers, voters, television watchers—are not really involved in the health care scene at this point in time. If they ever do become effectively involved, the degree of change now being forced upon us by DRG reimbursement and new Joint Commission requirements may seem minimal indeed to the degree of change forced upon us by those we presume to serve.

Image

The hospital industry presently lacks political support, public support, medical staff support, and employee support. In fact, at a weekend joint retreat, participants may identify the hospital's *image* as the most pressing issue, because it relates so directly to both economic and legal pressures on the hospital.

Example of the image problem—an excerpt of a letter from a friend not involved in health care . . .

> Because I know the kind of work you do, I thought you might be interested in my experience when I was in our hospital lately for a relatively minor problem. It seemed to me the nurses and other personnel were very involved in what they had apparently been told was their work, but very little of their work seemed to relate directly to the patient.

For example, at a time when my wife and I have given several thousand dollars over the years to the hospital (our names appear under "benefactors" on the plaque in the main lobby), it was a little discouraging to find that when I needed a wheel chair I was told there just weren't enough to go around. Yet we have a nice new awning out in front, automated bed rails, and plastic disposable dishes.

I tell you, Dick, I'm afraid our hospital has turned into the image of what some administrator thinks a hospital ought to be.

CHAPTER 6

From a buyer's market to a seller's market— just the beginning

The basic root cause of new pressures on the hospital management/medical staff working relationship is:

> **Physicians and hospitals alike, long accustomed to functioning in a seller's market, are now being forced to function in a buyer's market.**

As Thomas Frist, Jr., M.D., president, Hospital Corporation of America, says, "The mood in America . . . what is expected of the healthcare system . . . has shifted from *more* is better to more *efficient* is better."

Some healthcare professionals are reacting immaturely to the industry's cost-containment measures. Hospital executives and medical staff members are finding incredible ways to increase their own vulnerability by taking actions they mistakenly believe are protective. Ill-concerned, poorly thought out, short-term reactions are basically the result of panic. Not panic in just the economic-crash sense, but in the personal sense as well.

For Hospital Executives

As a hospital executive, you have been trained that boards of directors evaluate managers on the basis of how much growth they achieve. Now you have to forget growing and diversify just to *survive*. Achieving growth instead of entrenching and protecting what you already have requires fundamentally different attitudes and skills. A recent cartoon on the business page of a major newspaper shows a middle manager standing in front of the president of the company, with a declining-profits curve on the wall in the background. The president is saying, "Smedley, you were a great quarterback for the offensive team, but what we need now is defense."

Result: Panic!

For Physicians

Most physicians felt, until recently, that the next stop after training was to go to one or more hospitals and say, "Hi, lucky. I've chosen you!" The expected response was a welcome with open arms, and the kind of consideration that might lead one to believe that he or she had somehow transcended mortality.

Now, when the physician asks, "May I be on your medical staff?" the reply is, "Well, maybe. Who's your lawyer?" or "Don't call us, we'll call you."

Result: Panic!

Some hospitals and medical staffs are discovering new value in cooperative efforts. But in other hospitals:

- Hospital management is "restructuring" for the purposes of diversification and discovering new sources of revenue. Medical staff involvement in this process has been judged unimportant. Medical staff is saying, "Just when we began to have real input by having physicians on the hospital board and the chief of staff as an ex-officio board member, they sidestep us by creating 'super boards.' They don't really want medical staff input. Maybe the medical staff should have its own legal counsel."

- Hospital executives are aware that their future potential may be found by joining or forming a multi-hospital group. But the board is being sued by the medical staff who say, "Wait! You're not giving *our* hospital away!"

- While the medical staff accuses its hospital management of unfair competition, a full-page ad appears in the local medical society journal, inviting physicians to send their patients to a private radiology group—*not* to the hospital—for computerized tomography (CT scanning).

- At a time when proven accountability for cost, quality, and accessibility of care is the key to marketing *and* the conscience of cost-cutting, a hospital-wide accountability system is considered a very low priority by the medical staff and the chief executive officer.

> Hospital managers and medical staff members who have paniced, knee-jerk responses to each other's initiatives will find themselves with the disadvantage of the competitive wedge, rather than the advantage of the competitive edge!

Take the Long-Range View

Today's medical staff should react by trying to anticipate and head off ever-expanding pressures. The medical staff should expect:

- Heavier pressure from the government, insurance companies, industry, and the public to contain healthcare costs.

- Pressures to be accountable to patients and families to come from the Joint Commission on Accreditation of Hospitals (JCAH), labor unions, and the desire to be competitive—to be a "preferred provider" in marketing.

- Pressures to contain costs, *or* to be accountable to patient and family concerns, *or* both, *or* neither, to come from politicians, depending on which way the wind is blowing.

- The Tax Equity and Fiscal Responsibility Act of 1982 to be the first step to permanent sweeping changes in Medicare and, perhaps by implication and spinoff, in the entire United States healthcare system.

- The DRG (diagnosis related groups) system to someday be considered the primitive forerunner of a system that better balances clinical reality and economic necessity. Look for such a system to be the result of *joint* efforts of data processing specialists, clinical practitioners, hospital managers, payers, and perhaps even public representatives and government.

- A decline in the number of free-standing community hospitals and in the number of free-standing solo practitioner doctor's offices.

- A redefinition of the word "hospital" and more penetrating questions by hospital boards than, "Were all our beds full this month?"

- Resentment, turf-guarding, arbitrarily restrictive regulation, and unfair competitive practices to assure the immediate and long-range future of many attorneys.

- Changing management styles. Secretive, Machiavellian, manipulative styles will prove less successful than more open, accountable styles of management.

- The economic collapse of some hospitals directly traceable to inability or refusal to recognize the importance of developing a base of support for the hospital, among the medical staff, among the community served by the hospital, and in the political arena.

- Other hospitals to injure themselves through an over-zealous interpretation of competition. A football team doesn't win if its competitive strategy is so fierce that it has its own offensive line stand up, turn around, and tackle its quarterback.

CHAPTER 7

What has the federal government done to the hospital/physician relationship?

Some appear to believe the DRG-payment method, the question of limiting medical staff membership, and other new hardball issues, will automatically damage the hospital administrator/medical staff relationship. Nothing could be further from the truth. One thing that's certain is that the relationship will be different—hospital reorganization surely now will encompass the medical staff as well. A profusion of medical staff committees will give way to responsible clinical departments and individuals as the working units of the medical staff.

Medical staff/management structure and relationships will more directly acknowledge the mutual risk that physicians and hospitals share—economic and legal risks, but also image and ethical risks. There's never been a better opportunity to oil up and get some movement going at the rusty joint of medical staff-hospital relations. If that relationship is worse one or five years from now, it will be easy to blame the federal government. But medical staff members will have only themselves to blame for failing to take advantage of new attitudes and new responsiveness. Here's just one example. In the May,

1983, *Journal of the Illinois State Medical Society*, the "President's Page" by Robert P. Johnson, M.D., is entitled, "Medicine's Front Runners: The Positive Futurist." Dr. Johnson concludes:

> The positive futurist M.D. will learn to forecast events, plan for contingencies, prepare personal blueprints, anticipate a reconfiguration of medical practice, and stay flexible. These skills will enable him or her to meet the challenges of medicine in the decades to come.

This is written by a leader in organized medicine, a private practitioner of obstetrics-gynecology, in the pages of the same journal that only a year or two ago spoke of the insensitivity of those who would market the hospital's product to the consumer.

Now, leaders of both organized medicine *and* the hospital industry are likely to be more aware of their dependence on each other—to accept that it simply can no longer be "business as usual" in the healthcare field.

Secret Weapon of the Preferred Provider

In that environment, the hospitals and physicians *most* disadvantaged in these competitive cost-cutting times—those hospitals making the biggest error that can be made—will be those who automatically accept the assumption that the government has harmed the chief executive/board/physician relationship.

The one thing the Federal Government *has* done is fix it so that the relationship will not be the same in one year or five as it is now. There will be movement at this rusty, squeaky joint between the medical staff component of the hospital organization and the rest of the hospital, but that's not all bad. Some of us, who for several years have been looking for ways to get that stiff joint moving, welcome this opportunity.

Many hospitals are preparing to forge ahead rapidly with a new understanding of medical staff bylaws as a useful, day-to-day, management tool, not just a negative, legalistic document to be brought into play when there is a problem. And, in an increasing number of hospitals, new kinds of mutually beneficial, organizational relationships between doctors and hospitals are being explored. These hospitals have discovered five major keys:

- Responding to the need to compete, while not getting confused about who's "us" and who's "them."

- Responding to new reimbursement rules, in a way that can trim fat and duplication from healthcare costs, without assuming this can only be done by cutting quality.

- Success in marketing depends upon realizing that the dramatic change in healthcare is from "more is better" to "more efficient is better."

- Developing public and political support through projection of a positive image.

- Establishing the long-range view of goals and priorities so necessary to stabilize and protect the present stage of development of the private medical and hospital community.

It Won't Be Easy

The joint efforts described above must be established from a starting point of people with management backgrounds who have only two speed settings—fast run and sprint, and a medical staff which accepts change and innovation at only two speeds—slowly and not at all. They must be accomplished in the face of a diversity of opinions about the wisdom of such activities as restructuring, joining or forming a hospital group, diversifying and offering new services, recruiting in some areas of the staff while limiting other areas, and, depending on long-range plans, are based on a variety of assumptions that may or may not be correct now, and will almost certainly undergo change in this unstable era.

It won't be easy, because hospital administrators are defensive about people talking of the hospital glut, just as physicians are sensitive to discussions of physician surplus. (My wife, Joan, wants to know, "If there's such a doctor glut, how come here in Elmhurst, Illinois, we still have to wait two months to get an appointment?")

No one ever said it was going to be easy. But it may not be as difficult as it sounds either, if we are willing to acknowledge and learn from some errors we've made in the recent past.

One Error to Avoid: Continuing to Believe That Commercial Industry and the Hospital Industry Are Exactly Analogous

Santayana did *not* say that history *repeats* itself. What he said was, "Those who refuse to learn from history are destined to repeat its mistakes." That's a much less fatalistic statement. Ronald Reagan apparently believes it. During the furor over then-candidate Reagan being briefed with some of candidate Jimmy Carter's material prior to their pre-election debate, a political cartoon depicts Mr. Reagan thumbing through a manual entitled, "How Not to Handle It" by Richard M. Nixon.

Hospital executives and physicians would do well to take to heart a basic flaw in our thinking as hospitals have been forced to become more and more businesslike in recent years.

A working relationship of mutual trust and respect between hospital executives and professional staff is necessary because no pure control model or pure collegial model adequately encompasses the coexisting prerogatives of those responsible for managing the institution, and those responsible for managing patients.

PART III:
The Third Key:
We Know the Similarities
Between Hospitals and
Commercial Industry;
It's Time to Talk About
the Differences

CHAPTER 8

The reality of a hospital: decisions about managing the institution and individual patients

The correct organizational model for today's modern, complex hospital must reflect these facts:

- In a hospital, executives and policy makers are fulfilling their responsibilities by making decisions about the management of the entire institution.

  Simultaneously, individuals are making clinical decisions which, taken together, comprise the medical management of an individual patient.

- Sometimes these two types of decisions, institutional management and patient management, rest with the same individual. For example, the hospital pathologist is administratively responsible for part of the institution—his department—and is simultaneously clinically responsible for patient-care activities such as the accuracy of anatomical pathology reports and laboratory studies.

- And in such departments as nursing, institutional and patient-care decisions may be synonymous. For example, nursing policy and procedure manuals, a major tool in administering patient-care units, are (supposed to be) based on sound principles of clinical nursing.

But usually, the two kinds of decisions are not synonymous. For example, the hospital board, executive staff, and medical staff leaders will arrive at a policy decision to maintain facilities for open-heart surgery. But this policy decision is not useful in establishing which specific patients are appropriate candidates for such surgical intervention and which patients are not.

> A hospital usually experiences difficulty, and so may its patients, if management/policy decisions are made without input of those with clinical expertise and knowledge of day-to-day needs in the care of individual patients.

Example: Constructing a building or addition to house patient-care services certainly comes under the heading of institutional management. But, for various reasons, smart management seeks and heeds input and comments on architectural design from doctors and nurses who will be providing patient-care services.

> Only recently are physicians appreciating the truth of the corollary — individual clinical decisions can make a great impact on matters

related to financial stability and management of the hospital.

Example: The big example now, of course, is DRG payment. The thoughtfulness with which diagnostic studies, drugs, blood, and other patient services are "ordered" by physicians is the major key to retaining quality clinical decision making, and simultaneously protecting the financial viability of the health-care institution.

Physicians who back away from the details of DRG-based reimbursement, for whatever reason, may be doing their patients a disservice. Hospital executives who do not help medical staff officers establish educational programs explaining the nuances of DRGs *on a level* and *in terms* physicians can accept are doing the medical staff a disservice.

CHAPTER 9

Progress toward understanding

Hospital executives and managers may wish that physicians would understand that clinical decisions can no longer be made without considering their economic and legal consequences. Meanwhile, physicians may wish that hospital management would understand that economic decisions cannot be made in hospitals without considering their clinical and ethical, as well as legal, consequences. But wishes aren't enough. They never were.

The two biggest blocks to mutual productive effort so far have been:

1. Failure of clinicians who are members of the hospital's medical staff to appreciate their *dual* responsibility—to their patient and to the hospital to which they bring their patients for care.

2. Failure of hospital management to implement the corporate structure with full acknowledgment of a responsibility to the clinical decision makers and their patients.

Most members of the healthcare team are beginning to understand the responsibilities of this dual role. The executive staff must draw a circle and be sure it includes and surrounds the medical staff.

The Hospital Board

The hospital board was the first component of the hospital organization to understand its dual role—thrust upon it by law. A few years ago, hospital board members would have described their obligation as unidimensional—financial solvency for the hospital. Now, hospital boards are required by law to find effective ways of accepting responsibility for qualifications and performance of the hospital's professional staff as well. And lay board members *are* learning how to play this role effectively (see Part V—Specific Suggestions).

Nursing

Nurses can certainly explain to you the necessity (and frustration) of accepting a dual role. As hospital employees, nurses have one line of responsibility through supervisors and the administrator of nursing services, and they are expected to comply with relevant personnel policies applicable to all hospital employees.

But nurses are also in the thick of the clinical decision-making process, expected to be the primary respondent to the doctors' entries on the patient's order sheet, and to be responsible for certain independent nursing tasks to meet individual patient and family needs.

Healthcare executives and medical staff members would do well to understand current issues important to nursing, to consider these issues of high priority, and to move to respond to them so as to avoid counter-productive turf-guarding and internal dissension.

Administration

Some hospital administrators have a thorough understanding of their dual role. These hospital administrators handle the title "President" with great care, and have the respect of *both* their board and their medical staff. They have leadership instincts that make them highly valued, trusted, and respected confidants to medical staff and board.

Other administrators/executives attempt to apply the strict "power model" of executive leadership. These administrators assure their own failure since neither the board nor the medical staff will be convinced that the chief executive officer (CEO) considers seriously their needs or their suggestions for improvement. They shut out the medical staff—or give the impression they do, which comes to the same thing. This CEO has not grasped the concept of needing to function as a business executive in one sense and a sensitive health professional in another—always subject to the board of directors, but responsive also to the expressed needs of the clinical decision makers in the hospital.

The Medical Staff

Physicians fully understand their responsibility to their patients. But many medical staff members appear to have difficulty accepting the fact that when they bring their patients to a hospital for care they assume a *dual* responsibility:

- To their patient.
- To reasonable hospital/medical staff rules and regulations necessary to make the hospital's services available to and somewhat standardized for *many* physicians and *many* patients.

Take a look at figure 9-1 which is, believe it or not, an actual order sheet from a patient's medical record. To understand the underlying scenario, you must know that "Mr. Blank" is the CEO of the hospital.

Figure 9-1

PHYSICIAN'S ORDERS

		_____ HOSPITAL
		Drug Allergies:
		Diagnosis:
MR. ROBERT	☐ ANOTHER BRAND OF DRUG, IDENTICAL IN FORM AND CONTENT, MAY BE DISPENSED UNLESS CHECKED.	
① Transfer to Mr. Blank's care		
② Humidifier		
		_____ HOSPITAL
		Drug Allergies:
		Diagnosis:
	☐ ANOTHER BRAND OF DRUG, IDENTICAL IN FORM AND CONTENT, MAY BE DISPENSED UNLESS CHECKED.	
		_____ HOSPITAL
		Drug Allergies:
		Diagnosis:
	☐ ANOTHER BRAND OF DRUG, IDENTICAL IN FORM AND CONTENT, MAY BE DISPENSED UNLESS CHECKED.	
NURSE OR WARD CLERK		DOCTOR

In this case, the physician advised the patient in his office that she would have to be admitted to the hospital, and that the nature of her illness required placement in one of the hospital's special care units. The patient objected, stating that she wanted one of those private rooms on the side of the hospital overlooking the lovely park.

The physician acquiesced and requested that accommodation from the hospital's admission office, even though this general medical surgical unit was neither staffed nor equipped to care for the patient's specific medical problem.

When the nurses received the patient on this general medical surgical unit, the nursing supervisor reasonably advised the admitting physician that placement in the special care unit would be preferable. She was told, with implications of threatened job security, that she should just take care of the patient and not interfere with the doctor's business.

The supervisor persisted in seeking appropriate placement for the patient by notifying the administrator of nursing services, who contacted the CEO. The CEO asked the chief of staff if he would please intervene and explain to the physician the problem he was causing the nursing staff. The chief of staff refused to become involved, stating that he and the physician were good friends, that they refer patients to each other, and that he did not wish to jeopardize either their personal *or* professional relationship.

Left no alternative but to handle the matter himself, the CEO contacted the attending physician, explained the nursing staff problem, and requested that the patient be transferred into the special care unit. The attending physician, now furious at so many interruptions about this one patient, advised the CEO to mind *his* own business (which the CEO was) and again the physician threw in some threats of job security and a couple of cracks about "top-heavy management" with nothing better to do than interfere with rightful decision-making prerogatives of physicians. At this point, the CEO, having exhausted all remedies available to him, transferred the patient to the special care unit. The attending physician was so furious at this action that he then wrote the order, "Transfer my patient to the care of Mr. Blank" (Figure 9-1).

This incident is not an extremely unusual horror story. In fact, it's a fairly common example of the need to start at square 1 to develop and clarify an understanding of who's in charge of what at the hospital. Hospital managers don't write on order sheets, but they must insist that individual-practitioner behavior does not disrupt hospital routine. Individual clinical decision-making prerogatives of the medical staff do not extend to single-handedly changing or violating hospital policies and guides lines established for good reasons. It's the old story: Tony's Pizza Parlor doesn't cash checks; the bank doesn't make pizza.

By the way, there's a humorous ending to the "transferred patient" incident. A few days later, the CEO heard that the physician was now rather embarrassed over his handling of the situation. The CEO then asked the physician to come by his office, where the doctor said, "I guess you want to talk to me about that stupid order I wrote the other day." The CEO, reading this response as "enough said" said, "You bet I do. From now on, I don't mind you transferring a patient to my care, but when you do, you must have confidence in me. I called you in to tell you: don't you *ever* order a humidifier on one of *my* patient's again!" The CEO managed to ease the tension while emphasizing the relevance of and necessity for (at least some) hospital rules.

That's Progress Toward Understanding

For awhile, hospitals seemed to have progressed beyond the understanding of practitioners, policy makers *and even* trained hospital management professionals. But now, the rigid, "hospitals-are-like-any-other-industry" approach of the 1970s is abating. CEOs now know that limiting their attention to financial and legal concerns to the exclusion of professional concerns is no way to lead a successful hospital in the 1980s and 1990s. And *many* physicians are now beginning to understand the hospital as an organization and their place within it. Specifically:

- CEOs of successful institutions are paying attention to what their *professional staffs* suggest are important issues as well as to what their financial and legal advisors say are important issues.

- Many medical staff executive committees and hospital boards hold annual joint retreats for the purpose of educating each other and discussing common problems.

- Many hospital boards now claim physicians as full voting members.

- In addition to physicians as board members, the elected chief of staff is often an ex officio member of the board and is expected to represent medical staff interests and concerns to the board.

- Medical staff members are members of key committees such as long-range planning.

- In some hospitals, board members sit on relevant medical staff committees, such as credentials and the quality coordinating council.

- Boards of directors that evaluate chief executive officers (a still-emerging skill and activity) evaluate the CEO on ability to work with the medical staff, as well as ability to keep the hospital in the black.

- Some hospitals have established a "No Surprises Council"—an informal opportunity for representatives of the board, medical staff, and administration to learn more about each other's activities.

That's the good news.

The bad news is:

- Much remains to be done. For example, effective medical staff organizational function, with the grass roots medical staff member *really* feeling involved, is still the oddity rather than the rule.

- The recent advances in the board/CEO/medical staff relationship are now threatened by new pressures—cost-per-case payment and competition—that could cause a recurrence of distrust and suspicion.

> The remainder of this book is *not* devoted to continuing a re-statement of present problems and perspectives, but to specific suggestions, scenarios, and case studies that, while not necessarily palatable and easy to implement, are nonetheless necessary responses to new pressures and

threats to hospital managers, practitioners *and* patients, family members, and communities we presume to
serve.

PART IV:
The Fourth Key:
Facing Up to Reality

CHAPTER 10

Facing up to reality

Ever Hear of Old Copernicus?

Medical staff members and hospital managers whose joint efforts are successful in the 1980s and 1990s will be those who fully understand that new times will not simply allow new kinds of "initiatives" based on old assumptions.

What has recently happened in the American healthcare system is analogous to when the astronomer Copernicus came down from his telescope and told the people, "You know I've been studying the sun for years now, and I have to tell you . . . I don't think that sucker is going around us . . . I think we're going around it!"

The immediate reaction, of course, was denial, anger, frustration, and insecurity. Such a new assumption meant theories held for generations had to be changed. Suddenly, comfortable ways of thinking had to be discarded and new realities had to be faced.

DRG Payment

This system of paying for patient care has nothing to do with what we spend on the patient. It's not going around us anymore; we're going around it.

Medical Staff Composition

In the past, only "unlimited practitioners"—duly licensed physicians and dentists—could be on hospital medical staffs.

Now JCAH requirements that have long said, "A majority of the medical staff shall be physicians . . ." says that characteristics of an accredited hospital may include having practitioners—independently acting practitioners—on the staff if the hospital's bylaws say so.

In addition, JCAH insists that one characteristic of an accredited hospital is a new, more open management style in which the needs of the patients are better served by both individual and organizational communication between and among healthcare managers and practitioners.

It's not going around us anymore; we're going around it.

The Question of Quality versus Cost of Care

The healthcare system has gone from "more is better" to "more efficient is better." Technical capabilities are so amazingly complex and expensive that emotional issues like "rationing" patient care must now be genuinely considered, particularly in the midst of a *generally* constricting economy.

The American healthcare system isn't going around us anymore; we're going around it.

CHAPTER 11

Things are changing:
who will change them?

The American healthcare system was given numerous opportunities to face up to issues and problems caused by successes and advances in healthcare technology. Analyses of the reasons that many of those opportunities fell flat made interesting reading in the 1960s, '70s, and early '80s, but primarily produced a literature explaining why *everyone else* was at fault for not getting on with building a healthcare system suitable to patients, payers, providers, practitioners, purchasers, politicians, plaintiff's attorneys, and investigative reporters. Some of the excuses:

- It was all the American work force. The Dr. Spock babies of the 1940s, you see, had become the hippies of the 1960s and the middle managers of the 1970s. Their "me first," "not my job," and "your fault" turf-guarding attitudes permeated American society. Hospitals were no exception.

- New, more sound business and management practices had to be introduced into hospitals, you see. What can you expect a surgeon to know except surgery? Now, having recently been diagnosed as having a serious illness, I'm more convinced than ever that the "American healthcare system," whatever its managerial, consulting, data, and executive capabilities, boils down to a matter of the patient's confidence in an individual practitioner's commitment to working out individual patient-care problems.

- We simply came to do too much. It's difficult in educating physicians to teach them that "playing God" is to *withhold* an artificial, life-saving, manipulative device without also pointing out that in other situations the *application* of such a device might interfere with natural selection and other rules of nature.

- For whatever reasons, health care became a political football. Promising wide ranges of health care to an increasing number of federal and state beneficiary patients looked good in the eyes of the people, especially those who did not fully understand how government works. Election time promises must be backed up by votes when it comes time to spend the peoples' tax money.

- It was all the fault of organized labor, you see. They did such a good job of negotiating healthcare benefits that they put the pressure on the profit margins of American companies that could scarcely stand the strain, especially when foreign competitors seemed to be invading increasingly large percentages of American commercial goods markets.

- The era of mass communications and investigative reporting was all to blame, you see. Reporting positive news neither sells newspapers nor follows the investigative reporting parameters of always leading the newscast with the blood and the flames.

- And, of course, as Shakespeare said, "Let's kill all the lawyers." If we just didn't have to make a legal issue of everything, we could get on with the real business at hand . . .

You have heard that litany before. You can add to it, or subtract from it, or modify it. But the point is there for all to see.

> **We have been a nation of position-takers trying to fix the blame on someone else, instead of accepting our share of the responsibility for fixing the problems.**
>
> **It turns out that the only way to try to solve problems without admitting that we are part of the problem is to accept assumptions and suggest problem solutions that really do not compute.**

Administration	Medical Staff
Management says, "Doctors may be on the board, but are not there to represent medical staff interests."	But when the medical staff says, "We don't have enough medical staff input into board decisions," administration says, "But why not? There are three doctors on the board."

The government says, "Practitioners and institutional providers must make hard decisions about which patients get costly procedures or special care."

"Trust us," say both medical staff managers and practitioners. "We have a mechanism called 'informed consent' by which we attempt to provide the patient enough information to make a truly informed decision about whether or not they want to undergo or forego a treatment or an operation that may have significant consequences."

Medical staff members and hospital managers say, "Lawyers have too much power these days. They're into everything."

Ditto for consultants.

Practitioners say that cost in healthcare cannot be cut without cutting services to patients.

The government also says, "Don't exercise your judgment. Don't have go/no go criteria in dealing with small infants requiring expensive, high-risk care. Follow the Baby Doe law and don't play God by withholding available artificial life-saving measures."

The President's Commission on Malpractice concludes that, *as implemented,* the informed consent mechanism looks more like it is designed to protect doctors and hospitals from lawsuits than it is to provide the patient with needed information.

Medical staff members and hospital managers say, "A conflict?! I don't want to touch it. Call the lawyer!"

Ditto for consultants.

But there is a special view of a hospitalized patient. Even if a patient is only recuperating in the hospital following an operation, something must be done, it seems, to justify the hospitalization. For example: A patient at home on three meals a day would simply be going about the activities of daily living. For some reason, a patient in the hospital must have a total battery of electrolytes and a complete blood count drawn every morning in order to be sure that these ordinarily taken for granted bodily functions are recorded on pages and pages of laboratory results, with the information seldom used to make any adjustments in the hospitalized patient's care.

"Don't worry," says the CEO to the medical staff. "We're paying attention to practitioner and patient needs in the design of the new building. We have doctors on the building committee."

But when construction has begun and cost overruns are obvious, cuts and changes in building plans are made unilaterally by "the management team" without further consultation with either (a) the building committee or (b) individual practitioners with relevant clinical expertise who will be using that area of the building in which to care for their patients.

A physician complains, "Why don't administration and the board ever ask me for my ideas?"

When a solicitous administration and board asks this physician for his opinion, the physician says, "You're always wanting my free time. I don't really have time to give you an answer. Even if I did, you wouldn't understand it, because only doctors really understand patient care."

Nurses say, "Neither physicians nor administrators have enough respect for us as committed professionals."

Some of the same nurses say, "When it is time to be committed professionals, we will be committed professionals; when it is time to organize and strike, we will organize and strike; when it is time to view our problem in the light of feminism, we will take that approach, too."

"Hospitals are different now," say hospital managers, government, consultants, and others. "The real idea is to keep people well rather than to spend all our time taking care of the sick."

But I've just been diagnosed as having a giant cell tumor of bone requiring extensive surgery. Where do I go with that problem instead of a hospital? Who takes care of me instead of a competent practitioner?

Medical staff members and hospital managers say, "That new acute care center

Meanwhile, average waiting time in this hospital emergency room is 4½ hours.

that I didn't think would be much competition is doing better than I thought. I just don't understand it."

Average attitude in private physician's office is impersonal. (Several are saying that the success of new, free-standing patient-care services away from either traditional hospitals or doctor's offices represents a backlash against some of the traditional approaches of both practitioners and health-care institutional managers.)

Says the legislator or bureaucrat: "Healthcare is costing too much."

Says the same legislator, whose father has just been admitted to the coronary care unit: "For God's sake, Doc, mobilize this whole place and do whatever it takes!"

Medical staff leaders and hospital managers alike are saying, "We continue to be a professional, compassionate, caring institution . . ."

". . . but sometimes conveying the image that competition, entrepreneurial goals and being profit-making conglomerates are fun goals which we would sure like to pursue."

CHAPTER 12

Two simple keys to keeping control

Rediscovering the endpoint of productivity in a hospital

Patients, family members, payers for and purchasers of healthcare will not allow any definition of productivity in healthcare short of the best results. Perhaps it's as true in other industries, but the hospital industry in particular, in its efforts to respond to bureaucratic regulation, may have taken on the idiosyncracies, inefficiencies, and superficiality of those bureaucratic methods.

For hospital managers to work effectively with healthcare professionals, the priorities and job descriptions of healthcare managers are going to have to change

from:	to:
48% matters of legal concern	40% financial concern
48% matters of financial concern	40% professional concern

> 4% matters of   20% legal concern
> professional
> concern
>
> In other words, managers of health-care institutions are going to have to pay attention to what their *professional* staffs tell them is important, as well as to what their financial, legal, data, planning, marketing, and other consultants tell them is important.

The Cake Committee Approach to Keeping Control of the Private Healthcare System

Let's say that the American healthcare system is charged not with providing good healthcare to people, but with baking a cake. Practitioners of cake baking would say, "Well, let's go to the kitchen, bake a cake, establish parameters for excellence, present it to the people, have it evaluated, and have the job done."

But there is a feeling that management styles that have evolved in American hospitals, and perhaps other American industries as well, might take another approach. It might be too risky to just go to the kitchen and bake a cake. We might need, instead, to go through all of the following steps:

1. Appoint the Cake Committee.

2. Hire someone to staff the Cake Committee. Their title would obviously be "Cake Coordinator."

3. Establish the Cake Coordinator's office and system of files.

4. Do we have a written plan? Yes, we call this the recipe.

5. Good, then obtain legal review of the written plan before proceeding.

6. It will then be necessary, of course, to work with legislators to trade off statutes and regulations regarding the special interest group ("bakers") who may wish to negotiate legislative trade-offs in order to obtain an inside track on the cake baking positions at the hospital.

7. At this point, when someone asks, "Can't we just go to the kitchen and bake the cake now?" the reply comes back, "No way. We're too busy. We've got a lot to do now. We have to plan meetings and agendas of the Cake Committee, develop a confidentiality policy, establish minutes and contrived studies . . . Who has time to bake a cake?"

> In a stylized, not-too-far-fetched scenario viewed by some observers of the healthcare scene, activities seem more like a confused, mad-hatter's tea party than a clear and direct response to the nation's need for quality, cost effectiveness, and accessibility of healthcare services.

What This Has To Do With The Institutional Manager/ Practitioner Relationship

The Cake Committee approach often was the approach to implementing "risk management" in the 1970s. I don't know how many risk managers and hospital liability control experts have asked me, "Dr. Thompson, how can I get the doctor to come to my risk management committee meeting and participate in my risk management program?" Think about the question. The implication is: the important part of managing risks in hospitals is a committee meeting and a formal program fed by such contrived mechanisms as "incident reporting," and committee meetings and minutes as the ends, rather than effective individual communication.

It was heartening, in fact, just a few weeks ago to meet a person who is both an R.N. and an attorney, and who works with a hospital liability insurance program who said, "Of course. You're right. The reason incident reporting and other traditional mechanisms of risk management have not worked well in the past is that they have been designed to work *around* the physicians, rather than *with* and *through* them. Their emphasis has been programatic, artificial, and contrived, rather than a realistic effort to change attitudes and behavior of the physicians and other practitioners who of course are ultimately responsible for patient safety and, therefore, the reduction of hospital liability."

> The idea that patient risk can be managed in a committee has always been far too superficial to win the confidence or support of the physician or other healthcare practitioner.

> One key to restoring sanity to the American healthcare system is replacement of management styles with artificial, comfortable, non-threatening, non-risk-taking endpoints with management styles that challenge individuals to rediscover the acceptance of individual, personal responsibility for individual decisions and actions.

But That's Only One Key: Here's the Other One

> The other key to keeping control: mature practitioners who understand that their primary responsibility is to their patient, should also understand that when they bring their patient to the complex healthcare institution they assume a second obligation to co-workers and reasonable rules and regulations.

Many times, it seems that physicians do not know the difference between what an individual physician does and what the medical staff organization does. A personal complaint letter to the chairman of the hospital board of trustees is not "medical staff input." A medical staff organization exists and has, in the past, been ineffective in providing sufficient "medical staff input" not because the board and administration did not ask for it, in many instances, but because physicians were too immature or uncaring to make use of the existing organization.

Medical Staff Members Must Know and Understand What It Means to Agree to Abide by the Bylaws

Medical staff bylaws are a relatively simple document containing reference to only ten or twelve items (Figure 12-1). A clear set of medical staff bylaws should reflect the best thinking of the medical staff, board, administration, and hospital legal counsel and should be:

1. Protective of the patients and family members served by the hospital, including the medical staff component of the hospital.

2. Protective of the medical staff organization itself.

3. Protective of the rights and prerogatives of the individual medical staff member.

4. Protective of the hospital, in the sense of protection against corporate liability.

5. A clear and thorough explanation of the relationship between the hospital governing body, managers, and medical staff members.

The Major Problem

The major problem is that we are still seeking the right analogy to correctly describe the relationship between a hospital and its medical staff. We have tried the captain of the ship, and

Figure 12-1

MEDICAL STAFF BYLAWS ARE A SIMPLE DOCUMENT

1.   Name, Purpose

2.   Who may be appointed to the medical staff?

3.   How are they appointed?

4.   What may and must medical staff members do . . .

      a.   as medical staff members?
         (Vote, hold office, comply with reasonable rules of the hospital
         and/or medical staff)

      b.   as clinicians?
         (Clinical privileges)

5.   How is the medical staff organized to accomplish its functions?
    (Staff categories, departments, committees, officers, meetings)

6.   How does the medical staff deal with suspected marginal practice, disregard
    for rules, impairment, or disruptive behavior?

7.   How to amend?

8.   How to adopt?

9.   What protects an individual staff member's rights?
    (Hearing and appeals procedure; Fair hearing plan)

10.   Miscellaneous provisions.

that doesn't exactly fit. We have tried the 3-legged stool, and that is not exactly it. We have tried the unmodified corporate structure from commercial organizations, and that doesn't fit either.

> In today's world, where hospital managers and medical staff members are at mutual risk, economically, legally, ethically, and in terms of public image, an agreement by a medical staff member to abide by the medical staff bylaws means an agreement to abide by the board of trustees of the hospital. Until this is understood, none of the scenarios suggested in the final part of this book will assist the hospital in retaining control of its own affairs. *With* this understanding, the vicious cycle of invasive regulation and counterproductive in-fighting in hospitals can be broken.

How to Explain Medical Staff Bylaws to the Medical Staff

Hospital bylaws and medical staff bylaws are not opposing documents. With rare exceptions, hospital bylaws say that the board has fiduciary responsibility and authority for the affairs of the hospital. This is true both in terms of financial affairs and patient-care affairs. However, the hospital bylaws will state that since the majority of members of most hospital boards do not come from clinical backgrounds, the board chooses to delegate certain functions to its medical staff. These functions include such things as recommending to the board who should be appointed to the medical staff (based on a thorough examination of qualifications), bringing to the board's attention any issues related to marginal practice or disruptive behavior with an individual staff member, and performing professional reviews of clinical practice and providing periodic summary reports of these reviews to the board.

In most instances, the medical staff bylaws will essentially say, "Smart move. You're right. We have the expertise and interest. We accept." Then (see Figure 12-1), the medical staff bylaws describe, to the board's satisfaction, how the medical staff will accept this responsibility and self-governing authority.

> The medical staff that understands the concept of medical staff bylaws does not spend its time complaining about inadequate medical staff input, but spends its time finding effective mechanisms of implementation by which the provisions and intent of this continuum of hospital and medical staff bylaws become reality. Thus, instead of the Disneyland of the 1970s in which medical staffs fought boards and administration for control

of hospitals, medical staffs, hospital boards, and institutional managers can restore productivity, sanity, and self-control to the American health-care system.

CHAPTER 13

A prediction: a new set of management buzzwords

In the 1970s, a common phrase was "the system is the solution." If we could just find the right data processing system, method of obtaining and displaying "hard data," the right "corporate structure," and other structural solutions to our problems, we would have it made. By the end of the 1970s, the results of such a search were buzzwords like "economic survival," "fear," "over-regulation," and "decreased productivity."

In order to implement effectively the scenarios suggested in the final section of this book, you will find that the new set of management "buzzwords" and precepts you will need will relate more to use of problem-solving skills and interpersonal relationships than to the seeking of an automatic, canned, off-the-shelf solution to your problems.

*Time Spent Understanding Another's Viewpoint
and Helping Others Understand Your Viewpoint
is Productive Time Indeed*

Often, two people or two groups argue although they don't disagree. Think about it. A debate begins before terms are defined. This situation is called a "misunderstanding." The tragic outcome of the traditional "misunderstanding" is that clarification and communication never occur, and a mutual working relationship and agreement are never reached. The more hoped for result is for necessary definition to occur and success to be achieved.

> It may help you to keep perspective if you realize that all "situation comedy" is based on "misunderstandings."

Go Back to Square 1

In some hospital situations, a mutual working relationship never develops because either the medical staff or administration thinks, "It's no use to talk to them about that. We tried to before. They didn't pay any attention to us. In fact, they told us then that they didn't have time to discuss it. Why try again?"

Try again. Because:

- Attitudes and opinions change for the better for a variety of reasons.

82

- A major change in circumstances always makes it worth going back to square 1 and rediscussing specific issues. (Again, think of the switch from retrospective reimbursement to prospective payment by the DRG system — questions of limiting the medical staff and credentials issue — new, more functional Joint Commission requirements — it's not going around us anymore, we're going around it.)

Take the Initiative

Go ahead. Swallow hard and be the one to suggest going back to square 1. You may just solve a problem.

Example: A common conventional luncheon setting is round tables with eight people at each table. One usually gets seated with no more than one or two acquaintances, with the rest of the people at the table strangers whom one wishes to impress. In that situation, however they do it, if pie is to be placed for dessert, the pie is always placed equidistant between two dinner plates. That means that while you are trying to impress these strangers, unless you are an expert on etiquette, you must decide whether to take the piece of pie on your left or on your right.

At one such banquet, where all of us were obviously puzzled but embarrassed to show our puzzlement ("Is this my piece of pie over here or is that my piece of pie over there?"), the problem was solved by an individual who took the initiative by taking the piece of pie to his right. Once that was done, we all reached out and did the same thing, and the problem had been solved. Without committee meetings. Without elections. Without bylaws. Without managerial principles. Just by taking the initiative.

Don't Overgeneralize

A medical staff cannot establish an effective working relationship with an individual hospital executive or board member if the medical staff members cling to views about what "all administrators" are like. Similarly, hospital presidents will have difficulty establishing strong working relationships with their medical staff members if they approach responsive and open minded physicians in exactly the same way they approach Dr. Trouble, Dr. Yesterday, and the Warrior Physician.

Enough said.

Distinguish Objectives/Goals From Methods Used in an Attempt to Achieve Those Goals

You've seen it happen a million times. Someone gets a bright idea. Everyone knows the anticipated, desired result. But in between the idea and achieving the result is a step called "selecting and implementing the effective, appropriate method."

If method A is selected, the desired goal is achieved and all goes well. But increasingly in recent years, it seems that we have stumbled over selecting proper methods. When a poorly selected method does not work, the usual course is to discard the original goal, rather than to evaluate our methods for proceeding toward what may still be a desirable goal.

Example A: "This hospital," says the physician, "expects too much of its medical staff members. We have too many committees. They meet too often. They produce pounds of paper and many studies, but no effective impact on what I'm interested in—patient care. I'd come to committee meetings if we ever started on time, if we ever accomplished anything, and if we wouldn't run on for two or three hours. But since all the things I've listed are problems, my conclusion is that medical staff functions, including review of tissue, transfusion, antibiotic, drug, and medical record review, utilization review, and departmental meetings are of no value whatsover."

Example B: A physician says, "Administration makes information handlers and support personnel available to provide the key decision makers on the medical staff with the kinds of information we need to effectively self-govern to the satisfaction of the hospital board. Thus, we have the respect of the board and administration, and do not have to complain about 'inadequate medical staff input.'"

Ask yourself: Are we Hospital A or Hospital B? If there is difficulty establishing a good working relationship with medical staff members, is it because:

- There really is no value in the good idea of effective medical staff self-governance, or

- Is it because we need to reevaluate and overhaul the methods by which the goal of effective medical staff self-governance is being accomplished?

> If I didn't know better, I'd swear that the programs in health, administration, and the whole field of management have completely ignored the difference between goals and methods.

—*Hospitals Are Us*
Robert R. Cadmus, M.D.
Teach 'Em, Inc., 1979

A Major Key: Learning to Restate the Question

> Some problems, the way we state them, truly cannot be solved. But often, the desired objective can be obtained by changing the statement of the problem and approaching it from a different angle.

Example: It's graduation night at the local high school. Everyone is in a jubilant mood. But at the beginning of the ceremony the principal throws a damper on the evening: "I would like to remind each and every graduate," he says, "that you will not—repeat—you will *not*—throw your caps into the air at the end of the ceremony. We had some eye injuries last year . . ." Now, anyone who has ever dealt with the adolescent age group as a teacher, physician, or parent recognizes the challenge which has just been established. Surely now at the end of the ceremony there will not only be joy, but also defiance as graduates' caps are hurled one after the other into the air—taking a position—showing one's independence, personal rights, and inability to be interfered with.

But this night, at the end of the ceremony, there is not a single cap thrown into the air. Of course the air is filled with a little of everything else! From beneath their gowns, the students obtain and strew confetti, paper streamers, balloons, etc. The problem is solved, and the mood is jubilant once again.

What happened here? Perhaps without realizing it, the students resolved an impasse simply by changing the statement of the problem.

> As long as the problem was stated,
> "How can we get the principal to
> change the school policy?" the answer
> was, "No way." But as soon as the
> students changed the question to,
> "What can we throw into the air
> instead of our caps?" not only was the
> impasse relieved, but framing a
> solution did not require a lot of
> committee meetings, or a lot of time.

Might the Same Thing Happen in the More Serious World of the Hospital?

Example: Hospital administration, board, and medical staff leaders were faced with a difficult problem. A general surgeon in this small community hospital accepts referrals from several general practitioners and family physicians with offices in neighboring communities. In order to foster his large referral practice, the surgeon invites referring physicians to assist him in the hospital's operating room *whether or not these physicians are members of the hospital's medical staff and whether or not they have clinical privileges to first-assist at surgery.*

Both hospital managers and medical staff leaders had reached an impasse in resolving this issue. They had attempted administrative and legal recourse through letters and heard back not from the physician, but from the physician's attorney, threatening legal action if any further steps were taken to infringe upon the rights of this practitioner and those who referred cases to him. After all, in this day and age that might even be considered restraint of trade (the attorney implied).

A solution was found when the problem was re-stated. Rather than working so hard on the problem, "How can we keep the surgeon from doing this?" the question was changed to, "Is there any way we could allow this practice?" Examination of medical staff bylaws revealed provisions for temporary privileges for patient-specific purposes. This bylaws provision, to the mutual satisfaction of hospital leaders, the surgeon, and the referring physicians, was utilized to allow patient-specific temporary privileges (with carefully defined restrictions) that allowed the hospital, physicians, and concerned patients to be involved in a "win/win" solution.

Perhaps there's hope

Note that in the graduating class story, the students solved their problem by changing the question. A graduating class in the turbulent, protesting 1960s might not have handled the problem so gracefully. They might have taken up a collection and hired an attorney to sue the school board in an attempt to get the school policy changed!

Wouldn't it be good if that example, plus the reasonable approach taken to the real, genuine hospital problem described above, indicated the advent of new management buzzwords and styles that emphasize the use of what we know how to do in problem solving and interpersonal relations, rather than simply assuming that the first approach to resolving any conflict issue must be an adversary stance.

PART V:
The Fifth Key:
New Practical Approaches

CHAPTER 14

Hospital economics 101 for doctors

The Temptation to Overexplain

Teach physicians the 101 course in hospital economics, not the advanced seminar. That's hard for sophisticated hospital executives to accept because they would like to get on with the more interesting, sexier issues and activities such as financial contracts with physicians, new forms of hospital organization other than a "double set of bylaws," identifying entrepreneurial physicians and merging economic interests with them, and working with chief finance officers, planners, and marketing specialists on diversification, restructuring, and other structural endpoint solutions that recently have become the designer blue jeans of the hospital industry.

Hospital executives are learning that their success in financial planning and marketing ventures depends partly on what they know about finance, planning, and marketing, and partly on the degree to which physicians understand that these new initiatives are necessary.

There is less need for physicians to understand the exact legalistic, statutory, and financial details of DRG payment mandates, than to

93

> understand the impact of this change on both:
>
> - The individual physician's practice
>
> - The importance of improving specific mechanisms of medical staff organization self-governance.

The Physician's Need to Know:
How Does All This Alphabet Soup Fit Together?

Explain Figure 14-1 to physicians, both one-on-one and in such forums as medical staff meetings and Joint Conference Committee sessions.

In any business equation, revenue generated is price per service times the number of times the service or product is delivered. A profit, break even, or loss statement is produced when costs are subtracted from revenue generated.

> The problem, doctor, is the tremendous disagreement between those *writing* checks for healthcare, and those *receiving* checks for healthcare. Federal and state government, private insurance companies, and industrial coalitions believe that quality healthcare can be provided for less. Hospitals, physicians, and other

Figure 14-1

HOSPITAL ECONOMICS 101

PRICE
VOLUME
COST

―――――――――――――

PRICE x VOLUME = REVENUE $$$*

	Profit	(P&L
REVENUE* — COST =	Break even	State-
$$$$	Loss	ments)

―――――――――――――

*$$$$ = NEEDED BY PAYERS TO PAY FOR
         HEALTH CARE

*$$$$ = NEEDED BY HOSPITALS/PHYSICIANS
             "PROVIDERS"
         TO STAY IN BUSINESS, LET ALONE
         HAVE CONTINUED DEVELOPMENT —

> "providers" tend to argue that cost can only be reduced if quality of services is impaired.

The basic point in accepting the new reality is for practitioners to understand that while they were trained in "more is better" for the patient, the basic issue in health care now is economics. Practitioners are expected to go from "more is better" to "more efficient is better."

Those who are determined not to put anymore dollars into the health care system have attacked all of the factors in Figure 14-1.

Volume

Professional Standards Review Organizations (PSROs) and "utilization review" programs of the 1970s were efforts to reduce costs of healthcare by reducing the volume of services provided. While this goal made sense, selection of methods was not accomplished with study and care, and results were disappointing. In the 1970s, the primary definition of utilization review was to shuffle average length of stay data one more way to try to illustrate cost saving in healthcare. This was one of the two superficial, artificial methods of accomplishing a goal that was relied on in the 1970s. In fact, average length of stay is too superficial a definition of almost any activity one can name. For example, I have an 18-year-old son. My son's name is Greg. Greg's girlfriend's name, this week, is Linda. Frankly, when Greg goes over to Linda's house, what happens while he is over there is much more important to all three of us than how long he stays. Think about it. Length of stay rarely is a valid indication of cost or quality.

So, believe it, Doctor, there have been efforts for a decade now to attempt to control healthcare costs through reducing volume of services. As we will see in chapter 15, more recent initiatives in controlling costs now make a truly effective utilization review program a very important facet of a mutual hospital business/quality patient care continuum to be identified, circumscribed, and implemented by individuals who are knowledgeable about both costs of healthcare and the necessity for maintaining the quality of patient care services.

Cost

The next piece of the puzzle, Doctor, is that those concerned with healthcare decided to provide incentives to the healthcare industry and to practitioners by establishing an environment in which shoppers for effective healthcare would seek out preferred providers. This competitive model gave rise to such alphabet soup as:

- Health Maintenance Organizations (HMOs). These organizations, with a standard membership and premium arrangement, allow individuals and/or industries responsible for employee healthcare plans to contract with healthcare environmental services and practitioners who are willing to establish the fact that they provide needed healthcare services in the most efficient manner possible.

- Preferred Provider Organizations (PPOs). Again, a combination of healthcare environmental services and practitioners is expected to compete with other similar units to successfully market and secure the business of such purchasers of healthcare as industrial coalitions and private insurance company plans.

- Independent Practice Association (IPA). This is another version of the competitive model. All of these forms of healthcare delivery differ from the past in that the old sequence of a patient picking a physician, a physician suggesting a hospital for care, the physician taking the patient to the hospital as the hospital's "customer," and therefore being the central consumer of care is now changed. (Remember, it's not going around us anymore; we're going around it.)

> Thus far, doctor, there is consistency. Economics 101 in healthcare is that those writing the checks have decided to provide strong incentives to eliminate any waste from the healthcare system.

The Final Blow: Price Fixing

The biggest buzzword in the healthcare industry at this writing is "DRG payment." This system of payment for healthcare and the legislative mandate by which it is implemented will have undoubtedly undergone innumerable changes, even during the production phase of this book. Thus, it's not the purpose of the following section to give a detailed description of either the diagnosis related group (DRG) data system or the Tax Equity and Fiscal Responsibility Act (TEFRA) and subsequent measures mandating this payment plan. The purpose is to point out that medical staff managers need to make the *impacts* of these new initiatives clear. The following are examples of some facts of life that physicians must be made to understand and accept. You will be able to add to, modify, and improve upon this list as time goes on, but the *approach* must be upfront. Relevant questions of physicians must be given an effective and honest response.

What is TEFRA?

Doctor, the Tax Equity and Fiscal Responsibility Act of 1982 is an omnibus bill, which affected many existing legislative statutes. The first thing that might be said is that TEFRA is the answer to the old 1970's question "What could possibly be worse than PSRO?" From 1965 through 1982, reimbursement for federal beneficiary patients was on a retrospective, budget-specific basis. In other words, the patient was treated and a statement or claim was submitted and honored by the government (following application of what most hospital finance people felt was an unfair reimbursement formula). In TEFRA, Congress directed the Health Care Financing Administration (HCFA) to begin basing payment for the care of federal beneficiaries on a limited, per case amount *irrespective of the amount of dollars spent in caring for the federal beneficiary patient.*

The thinking of Congress is clear: Social Security must be saved. Defense must be cut as much as possible and still stay defensive enough. Congress selected the healthcare system payment plan as a mechanism of freeing dollars for other purposes.

(NOTE! Hospital executives will note the "guts ball" involved in giving this straightforward explanation to the medical staff. Such logic will fall on deaf or suspicious ears when a physician sitting in a meeting hearing such heresy has just come from the bedside of an ill patient for whom he has been trained to "do whatever it takes" to make the patient well. This straightforward explanation is the medical staff manager's best hope for helping the physician understand that this is not the fault of hospital management, but of the combination of amazing, technological healthcare capability in a generally constricting economy.)

When Does This Go Into Effect?

This economic reality is not a future plan for which we have time to prepare. Most if not all hospitals in the country already are being paid for healthcare in this way.

Well, At Least It's Only Federal Beneficiary Patients and It's Hospitals Only

Wrong, Doctor. Industrial coalitions, Blue Cross, private insurance companies, and all who write checks for healthcare are moving as rapidly as possible to the "capped" payment system.

But This Doesn't Make Sense—Some Patients Have Heart Attacks and Some Have Strokes

Yes, the government knows that. Enter the DRG system of lumping patients according to length of time in the hospital and hospital services utilized. Whereas the TEFRA law simply says that a hospital will receive so many dollars per Medicare patient treated, DRGs make an effort to gear payment, at least somewhat, to the patient's medical condition and nature of treatment.

But Still: Some Heart Attacks Must Be Managed Differently From Others

The government knows that, too. Innumerable bureaucratic factors and appeals processes must be examined (the implementation of which will undoubtedly prevent this scheme from really saving any money in American healthcare). But, for the time being, the government's major argument is economic, not clinical. They understand that some heart attacks require more or less clinical services than others, but will take little time to argue with the clinician about fine clinical points. You will find that their bottomline argument is, "Over time, it will all even out. You will spend more on some patients and collect less; you will spend less on some patients and collect more."

What Does All This Really Mean?

The following analogy has helped many understand the brand-new ballgame faced by practitioners and hospitals assuming responsibility for patient-care results within a contracting economy:

If you own a woodframe house and you are contracting with a painter to paint the house, would you rather contract with the painter by the hour plus materials, or by the job? Remember that contracting by the hour plus materials means that if extra help is used on the job, there is delay completing the job, or paint is spilled on the job, the painter will simply include those costs in his or her statement to you, and you will pay for them. On the other hand, if you contract by the job, you will agree to a specific dollar figure and efficiency of the work will be up to the painter. There will, in fact, be incentives to complete your job as rapidly as possible, which can be a factor to your advantage.

Most people say that they would rather contract by the job than by the hour plus materials.

So would the government—from 1965 to 1982, the government con-

> tracted with healthcare professionals by the hour plus materials saying, "We trust you to do whatever it takes to give the best possible care to federal beneficiary patients."
>
> Now the government has changed its mind. The contract is by the job. "Finish the work—here is what the price list says the work is worth—here is your check."

But Whatever Happened to the Quality Care Question?

You're sharp to notice that whether one contracts with the painter by the hour or by the job the question of the quality of the paint job is not addressed. It is even more important to notice that when one contracts *by the job*, incentives may be introduced to complete the job in a hurry with even *less* attention to quality.

> The gamble of professional politicians is that cost cutting in healthcare and pressure applied to the healthcare system will be politically acceptable even to individuals who depend on the American healthcare system in time of personal need.

> Now no doubt exists that the TEFRA/
> DRG-payment mandate will reward
> either appropriate, efficient care for
> patients provided through the mature
> responses of institutional managers
> and practitioners, *or* the system will
> reward thoughtless corner cutting
> without genuine concern for impact
> on the healthcare needs of the popula-
> tion which a given healthcare institu-
> tion presumes to serve.

*The Physician's Basic Response: "The Government's Not
Going To Tell Me How to Practice Medicine"*

Freedom of choice in medical care is not necessarily dead.
What is dead is the system under which many of us trained
. . . complete freedom of choice at someone else's expense.

In order for practitioners to retain freedom of clinical decision
making and for hospital board members to retain freedom of
policy making and day-to-day managers to retain freedom of
management decisions, it is going to be necessary to face the
reality of accountability. If the healthcare industry's and practitioners' decisions are mutually thought out, free of duplication and excess cost, and in the best interests of the healthcare
needs of the nation, then it will not be necessary for the
government or anyone else to dictate our decisions.

If our decisions are not accountable, then it's a fact of life—
both institutional and individual clinical decision making *will*
be dictated.

The Vulnerable Ostrich

Perhaps this will all just go away. Don't believe it. The ostrich with its head in the sand has always looked to me like one of the most vulnerable creatures alive, with one of the most inefficient protective mechanisms ever devised by nature. DRG payment is *not* just another federal program that will be altered by a change in administrations. The real-world question is not, "How are we going to beat the system?" but "How are hospital managers and practitioners going to work together to respond maturely in a way that diminishes the negative impacts of this new threat?"

Effect on Medical Staff Functions

Hospital chief finance officers and medical records people will be assisting physicians with understanding that the accuracy of coding the face sheet of the patient record now actually impacts the size of the check a hospital will receive for services provided to federal beneficiary patients.

Hospital leaders will assist physicians in understanding that it is an inappropriate response to think that this is a problem of hospitals only. Whereas cost cutting with a vengeance has begun in the institutional area because most dollars are spent there, impacts on the size of the check received by physicians for certain services provided to federal beneficiary patients are already in effect.

The ripple effect of the DRG-payment plan will immediately include such factors as:

- *A tightening of the screws by the JCAH.* "Everyone else is talking cost," reasons the JCAH, "that makes us important guardians of quality. We are going to insist on genuine accountability systems in hospitals, rather than continuing to settle for fluff, busywork, contrived studies, and little impact in improving effectiveness and efficiency of patient care."

- *Temptations in planning and marketing that are going to be hard to resist.* There may be a tendency on the part of some hospitals to attempt to gear up for the highest paying types of patient, with little regard to being responsive to perceived and expressed healthcare needs of a total community.

- *Attempts at "getting around the system."* These will undoubtedly be thought of, and will be ill-advised. For example, it will occur to hospitals that total revenue is total discharges times dollars per discharge. Why not then just admit more people? In this respect, the Peer Review Organization (PRO) system (Did you notice the federal government decided *not* to get rid of PSRO?) is looked upon as one watchdog to prevent such fraudulent and abusive activity.

- *Tendencies for healthcare managers and practitioners* to waste time blaming each other for this turn of events. This tougher approach to hospitals and practitioners occurred because in the past neither organized hospitals nor organized medicine effectively provided evidence to dispute suspicions that neither patient management nor institutional management have been as effective and as cost effective as they could have been.

- *The ripple effect suspicion that some may not be willing to cooperate.* It's possible that those who would disrupt the private healthcare industry would enjoy being forced to take over the private healthcare industry because of in-fighting, turf-guarding, and the filing of lawsuits prevented the discovery of information-sharing and cooperative problem-solving efforts required to find a firm handle on this new situation.

CHAPTER 15

Examples of mature responses

Example 1

Proper Approach to the Medical Staff

Figure 15-1 illustrates the way in which the new economic facts of life were presented to the medical staff by a wise hospital manager. The reward is an effective, hospital-wide response that allows this small but sound patient-care institution to be well on its way toward being a survivor in today's environment.

Figure 15-1 was presented to the medical staff with the notation that the hospital was $96,000 in the hole for only the month of January 1983; this was the result of TEFRA and DRG reimbursement. The medical staff immediately asked how they could help. The defensive moves list was ready and was discussed, modified, and adopted by the medical staff.

Example 2

Overhauling UR Methods

Our concept of utilization review in the 1970s was too superficial. We felt that we could afford avoiding the issue of defining and describing cost and quality. The new economic facts of life allow medical staff members and hospital managers to

Figure 15-1

EXPLAINING PPS TO THE MEDICAL STAFF

Effective January 1, 1983, Medicare payment to ABC County Medical Center for inpatient care is based on $2,416 per Medicare admission.

Impact — January 1983

Actual   157 x $3,025 = $474,925
 157 x $2,416 =   379,312

Medicare Pay $ 95,613
Below Cost

Defensive Moves — Medical Staff

1. Emphasize preadmission lab and x-ray testing before admission — elective surgery cases.

2. Dismiss and readmit for cases where appropriate — delay for surgery.

3. Dismiss as soon as possible:
   Home Health
   Nursing Home
   Hospice (Future)

4. Write primary diagnosis on progress sheet at time of dismissal.

5. Overhaul U.R. program.

discover the relationship between cost and quality—it turns out we've been looking in the wrong place.

The relationship between cost and quality of healthcare services is easy to find if one looks at individual patient-care encounters, not at global explanations and complicated data-processing printouts (see Figure 15-2).

The relationship between cost and quality of care must be understood by both medical staff members and institutional managers.

For every patient with a medical problem, a wide range of services might or might not be ordered—ranging from administering blood, oxygen, or drugs to performing an operation. For each patient with each medical problem, each of these services is either indicated or not indicated. If the service is indicated and ordered, that is good quality care. If the service is not indicated and not ordered, that is good quality care in the sense of accountability to payers for care.

On the other hand, if we overreact to economic pressures and cut corners by avoiding ordering needed patient-care services, then we have a problem with accountability to the patient—a quality problem. If, on the other hand, we overreact in the direction of believing that we must do whatever it takes, thoughtlessly and copiously, then we may have a double problem:

- accountability to those paying for the services we are ordering without careful thought.

- the patient may not receive the best care possible because it is easier to thoughtlessly order a battery of laboratory and clinical services than it is to talk with, examine, and determine the genuine needs of the patient.

Figure 15-2

THE RELATIONSHIP OF COST TO QUALITY

	Ordered	Not Ordered
Needed	+	(—)
		(🚶 accountability) !!
Not Needed	(—)	+
	($ accountability)*	

The Dual Accountability of "Utilization Review"

* ● 1970's Emphasis,
  Due to Retrospective Payment Incentives — Related "Regs" & PSRO

* ● 1980's Emphasis,
  Due to Economic Survival

!! 1970's — Little mention

!! 1980's — May require surveillance *because* cost/case systems can "reward":
  ● Efficient, appropriate care

and ● Arbitrary cost cutting without reference to patient results/safety

  ● PPO's must offer more than $$ discounts (effective results)

Once this simple relationship between cost and quality is understood, new, sophisticated methods of utilization review will rapidly emerge to assist us in properly matching the use of ancillary services and patient needs.

For example, it is already possible to collect and calculate data by physician, by diagnosis, by procedure, and by hospital, that compares:

- AAC = Average Ancillary Charges
- ATC = Average Total Charges
- LOS = Length of Stay
- Patient Mix Data—So that it cannot be argued that discrepancies in utilization of needed services are explainable on the basis of the severity of illness of a patient mix.
- Quality Data—That appropriate use of ancillary services over an appropriate period of time produces the desired patient care result, without undesirable effects.

The reaction of several physicians to this overhauling of primitive utilization review programs in hospitals has already been that, "I didn't attend these meetings before because it was all for the government. All we did was shuffle length of stay data. But *this* looks productive!"

Also notice, then, that with that kind of reaction on the part of practitioner members of a hospital's medical staff, a chief financial officer (CFO) need not seek back-door, Machiavellian ways to try to deal with what I have heard one CFO refer to as "economic malpractice."

Example 3

A New Look at the Medical Staff Reappointment Process

Periodic reappointment to the hospital medical staff has primarily pursued the legalistic leanings of traditional approaches to medical staff bylaws. The new approach to medical staff bylaws is that the provisions of this document and the methods by which these provisions are implemented should be extensions of medical staff self-governance—useful day-to-day management tools—rather than simply administrative and legal recourses that must be used when recalcitrant individuals do not respond to reason.

The medical staff reappointment process will be valuable to us in these new economic times if we can use it as another example of getting rid of some attitudes that do not compute.

At one time, a medical staff member applied for membership and privileges on the staff and enjoyed these privileges lifelong. In more recent years, it has become routine for the medical staff member to reapply for a position at the hospital. Now, when we began this we explained to physicians that this was nothing to fear. After all, every employee of an organization such as a hospital undergoes an annual reevaluation. The reevaluation of the medical staff member, we explained, was exactly analogous.

> This is an example of not paying enough attention to the difference between an expressed goal and the choice of a method for accomplishing that goal.

The fact of the matter is that employees do not reapply for their jobs every year. The annual evaluation is an appraisal and feedback time. "This part of your performance is good; this part of your performance requires immediate improvement; this part of your performance is so outstanding that you're being commended for it." The employee, in other words, does not need to live in fear for an entire year of a time when a secure position is placed in unreasonable jeopardy. On the other hand, the legalistic approach to medical staff reappointment has been such that a medical staff member must watch his or her mailbox to see if reappointment has occurred and if so, if all current privileges have been renewed.

In addition, if we are completely honest about medical staff reappointment being analogous to evaluation of an employee, we should recall that the employee is involved in the evaluation. A face-to-face discussion is held, and an opportunity for give-and-take is established. Not so in the past with the reappointment procedure for physicians. This has been no problem to doctors because reappointment, so far, has been a rubber stamp. But as hospital managers, board members, and even medical staff leaders, more jealously guard increasingly limited positions on hospital medical staffs, the same objective, face-to-face discussion about performance—both quality and economic performance—will need to be held between and among medical staff and hospital leaders.

Figure 15-3 suggests one way in which such information might be tabulated and prepared for individual discussion with a medical staff member.

Figure 15-3

ACCOUNTABILITY FOR PATIENT CARE
Appraisal of Clinical Performance

(Includes patient results, utilization patterns, availability and attitudes)

Name _____

Specialty _____ Staff Member Since_____

Service Chief/Chairman_____ Date _____

☐ Mailed   ☐ Individual Discussion

Clinical Area of Practice	Data Source(s) Used	Evaluation		
		Outstanding	Acceptable	Improvement Necessary
Blood Utilization				
Drug Utilization				
Antibiotic Utilization				
Tissue Review				

Patient Results
  Infections
  Complications
  Mortality
  Patient's benefit
    from hospital care				

Patient's Medical Records
  Timeliness of completion
  Legibility
  Informational value				

Diagnostic Accuracy				

Figure 15-3 cont'd.

Clinical Area of Practice	Data Source(s) Used	Evaluation		
		Outstanding	Acceptable	Improvement Necessary

Utilization Appropriateness
  Admissions
    Number
    Appropriateness
  Length of Stay
  Patient Services
  Appropriateness
    Laboratory
  Radiology
  Rehabilitation
  Respiratory Therapy
Social Services
 	
_____
_____				

Consultations				
Incident Report Analysis				
Any Patient or Personnel Comments				
Attendance at CME Opportunities				
Other				

COMMENTS: _____

_____

by: _____

Title: _____

Chief/Chairman of Dept/Service

CHAPTER 16

Consequences of weak medical staff organization

In recent years, financial and legal restructuring of the hospital corporation has become a fine art. CEOs have responded vigorously and positively to urgings from their national organizations and legal and management consultants that such restructuring is imperative in response to new financial and legal issues.

But What About the Medical Staff Structure?

Paradoxically, one of the major underpinnings of the total hospital organization—a *professional* structure on which medical staff managers and practitioner leaders alike should be able to rely—was hardly even considered important in a total restructuring of the organizational picture of today's modern hospital.

The result is that medical staff leaders, patients, payers, the community, the hospital board, hospital employees (responsive to physicians through the order sheet), and others absolutely dependent on the physicians's central position as the coordinator of patient care, have almost universally complained of the unresponsiveness of the medical staff.

Just as physician leaders in hospitals have been mistaken to think a weak

> administration and board is protective of medical staff interests, so have some hospital board members and executives increased their vulnerability through a failure to take initiative in prodding the strengthening of a truly effective medical staff self-governance organization.

What Needs to Be Done

Take a look at existing medical staff bylaws through the eyes of effective organizational managers, not just adversary attorneys. (See Figure 12-1, chapter 12.) Notice that one of the questions answered in medical staff bylaws is, "How is the medical staff organized to accomplish its functions?" In the past, two basic approaches have been taken in building medical staff bylaws:

- "I'm a doctor who's always really been interested in medical staff bylaws. I will just write them for you. I don't really understand the distinction between what the general medical staff meeting does, what the executive committee meeting does, why we have to have both clinical departments and medical staff-wide committees. But I do know that the main purpose of the bylaws is to have a document on file to show the JCAH when they come. When the bylaws are ready, I'll let you know. Meanwhile, as I prepare them, I will build in as many of my own self interests as the medical staff bylaws committee, executive committee, and hospital board will allow."

- "Dear Dick: I'm the chief of staff of this hospital and we look forward to your coming to visit with us. You should know that we are revising our bylaws, but they're not back from the hospital lawyer yet."

Neither of these traditional approaches to building medical staff bylaws gave medical staff leaders an opportunity to really consider the organizational structure of departments, committees, and responsible individuals by which the medical staff could be self-governing, subject to the policies of the hospital governing body and necessary restrictions of the law.

Suggestion: Put a group of two or three physicians and a hospital administrator in charge of "professional affairs" to work drawing an organizational diagram of what your medical staff bylaws say. The reason is that such an exercise can turn a hodgepodge of words with legalistically described committees and functions into a clear trail of authority and information that relates the medical staff to the rest of the hospital. It then can provide—as much to the relief of hospital managers as medical staff leaders—an effective, responsive medical staff organization that, believe it or not, begins to take genuine pride in its role in hospital affairs. See Figure 16-1 for an example.

In this hospital, other organizational charts emphasize the details of administration, nursing, and hospital patient care departments. This particular diagram emphasizes a tie-in between the medical staff organization and the rest of the hospital through the "QCC"—the Quality Coordinating Council—which is a rapidly emerging model by which interests of practitioners, managers, hospital department heads, patients, and key personnel such as finance, medical records, and risk management, can be discussed.

The important part of the diagram is that this medical staff

Figure 16-1

MEDICAL STAFF ORGANIZATION: WORKING RELATIONSHIPS BETWEEN INFORMATION

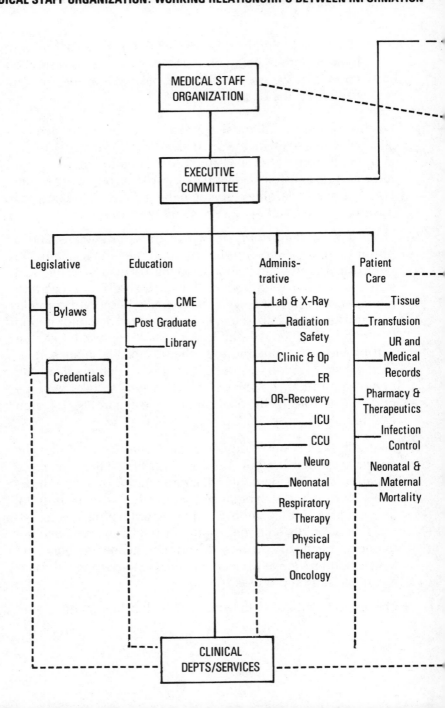

REVIEW, COMMITTEES AND DEPARTMENTS

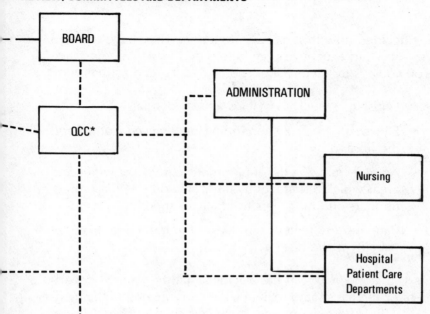

*Quality Coordinating Council

Reproduced with permission from Thompson, Mohr & Associates, Inc.,
P.O. Box 67, Elmhurst, IL.

has decided how they need to function. They have decided they need an executive committee, and its prominent place is obvious. They have divided medical staff organizations into:

- Legislative, such as bylaws and credentials.

- Education, such as continuing medical education and the library.

- Administrative, a list of numerous clinical activities and areas which require joint efforts of various kinds of practitioners and managers to manage smoothly.

- Patient Care, review activities—the traditional litany of "quality assurance" activities.

Next, this medical staff has decided that the clinical department or service should really be the working unit of the medical staff. Information and activities listed above should primarily be relayed to and acted upon at the departmental level.

A Surprising Note

This staff is to be congratulated on its clear thinking but might be surprised that they have not invented anything new. In 1917, the American College of Surgeons promulgated a one-page "standard" for hospitals. Among other things, this document stated that physicians practicing in the hospital should be organized into a definite staff and that the staff should meet monthly to transact its business. This document did *not* suggest that a large medical staff might wish to appoint various medical staff-wide committees. Rather, the document suggested that a large medical staff might wish to meet by department so that the clinical expertise and interests of practitioners in the hospital could best be utilized.

> Medical staffs that are rediscovering the clinical department/service as their primary working unit are successfully reversing the bureaucratic, non-productive impact of at least thirty years of requirements for diffuse, ineffective medical staff-wide committees.

Enter the New Breed: The Carefully Selected, Well-Oriented, Organizationally Aware Medical Staff Leader

So, you feel good now. You've discovered that medical staff bylaws can be viewed as a useful instrument. That's a great start, but now face the fact that you haven't yet accomplished anthing that is functionally an improvement over "the good old days."

> The next step—identify and cultivate the new breed—the physician leader who understands the proper use of organizational methods.

Who Wants to be Chief This Year?

The new look of effective medical staff self-governance begins with careful selection, orientation, and guidance of medical staff leaders. As most everyone knows, selection of such medical staff leaders as clinical chiefs of service has not been careful and thoughtful in the past. The usual scenario is: "It's annual meeting. Time to name a new chief of surgery. Who shall we select?" "I don't know. Charlie, when were you chief last?" "Charlie's not here. He's on vacation in Hawaii." "That settles it. I move the secretary cast a unanimous ballot for Charlie as chief of surgery for next year." "So moved and carried. Let's get on with the important business. Who's going to complain to the administrator about the nursing attitudes? They're questioning our orders again!"

Any good sports fan knows that a good team begins with recruiting. Thus, the result of the above scenario can be easily predicted. It is not twelve months of effective clinical service and department leadership in medical staff affairs. It is a lackadaisical monthly meeting at which a chief with no interest in the position routinely goes through the motions of reading an agenda prepared by an administrative secretary, with the primary purpose of creating the illusion that required medical staff functions are being fulfilled.

> Medical staffs that have invested neither the time nor the interest in establishing a good, self-governing organization have only made themselves vulnerable by leaving gaps that others—administration, board, insurance companies, Joint Commission, "the government," risk management, quality assurance, the nursing department, etc., have been only too happy to fill.

Suggested Responsibilities of Chief/Chairman of a Medical Staff Department or Service

Prior to introducing an individual's name to be clinical service chief, present medical staff leaders should sit down in private with the candidate to be sure that the importance of the position is clear. At least the following points should be discussed:

1. The *least important* task of a clinical service chief is to conduct a monthly meeting. If this book has not made anything else clear, it certainly should have clarified that the risky economic, legal, ethical, and image issues jointly faced by the hospital and the medical staff will *not* await a monthly agenda and a monthly meeting. Matters must be taken care of on the spot, day-by-day, by an individual who is willing to accept responsibility (with the full back-up of the continuum of hospital and medical staff bylaws, as described).

2. The chief of service is expected to be a coordinating point representing the viewpoint of his or her department and the medical staff to the board and administration, while at the same time accepting and relaying concerns of hospital management to those making *clinical* management decisions. We can no longer afford the ploy of selecting the most obstreperous, outspoken, troublesome physician to be a thorn in the side of administration and the board.

3. The responsible chief of service must be willing to stifle doctors' lounge talk of, "What are *they* trying to do to *us* now? *We* have no input." This individual must understand that he or she is the personification of the medical staff organization. Rather than complaining in

the doctors' lounge, the chief of service must orient medical staff members to provide the input and see that the input *is* provided.

4. The clinical service chief (or other medical staff officer about whom we are speaking) must be articulate. He or she will be expected to speak to:

    *   *Other clinical departments.* Frankly, the only resolution to such questions as, "Who recommends family practice privileges?" is dependence on the ability of two individuals—usually the chief of family practice and the chief of another department—to articulate issues and work together to resolve potential conflicts.

    *   *Medical staff-wide committees and the executive committee.* It is no longer necessary for medical staff members to think the only way to have organizational input is "one man, one vote" in a town meeting that occurs once a month at which intimidators and orators carry the day, and the semblance of democratic self-governance may be illusory at best. Physicians who understand effective ways to have input into organizations will discuss, debate, and decide their positions at the departmental meetings and depend on their articulate spokesperson—the chief—to make their wishes and concerns known to broader representative groups.

    *   *Co-workers.* Nurses especially have been frustrated for years that regardless of their best tactful efforts, individual physicians have not responded to concerns about illegible orders, possible medication errors, needs that patients express to nurses and that

nurses then attempt to relay to physicians, and respect for their training and ability. One of the major needs in American hospitals today is to work out some mechanism by which nursing issues are addressed. The responsive, articulate (but not "pushover") chief of a medical staff service is an excellent beginning in that direction.

- *Decision-making authorities outside the medical staff.* Obviously, selected medical staff leaders must be articulate and persuasive in dealing with the executive administrative staff of the hospital and the hospital governing body.

5. In the past, when a committee member has been asked, "When do you serve as a committee member?," the physician replied, "Well, once a month, when the committee meets, of course. When else?"

The well-selected, qualified, and oriented medical staff leader will now be expected to review information of all types and provide conclusions and recommendations on a day-to-day basis. Examples include, but are not limited to:

- Applications for membership and privileges to the staff, including new applications, renewal of present privileges, or requests for additional privileges.

- Incident reports—one of the major difficulties in many hospitals today is that the "incident reporting" track goes directly to administration's risk manager, even including incident reports that relate to practitioner performance. Hospital managers can never be expected to change that routine until effective medical staff leaders make themselves available to be interested in the evaluation of such reports.

127

- General patient-care information from quality assurance activities. The responsible physician leader, instead of just waiting for a monthly committee meeting, needs to assist information handlers and relevant authority individuals in deciding which information needs to go to which individual, which department meeting, or which committee.

- Evaluation of the institutional needs of a particular clinical department. What does the clinical service chief think of the staff adequacy and pattern of the qualifications of nurses and other employees working with his or her patients? Of the need to foresee replacement of an obsolete piece of clinical equipment?

- Advice/instructions/mandates that might be given to members of the chief's department by someone else. For example, a clinical service member reports that the CFO of the hospital has directly confronted him or her about a pattern of "economic malpractice." The clinical service chief must be ready to intervene to resolve the conflict.

6. The new breed of chief of clinical service is a counsellor/advisor/admonisher.

Medical staff self-governance now requires cognizance of and willingness to abide by reasonable hospital and medical staff rules, clinical performance concerned with patient *and* economic aspects of care, respect for co-workers, and acceptance of one's role as a member of a complex business/clinical management team.

Example: The importance of maintaining "peer" contact in resolving new issues is exemplified by the following statement:

> Hospital managers are rapidly learning that one will never, never, never get a practitioner voluntarily to change ordering habits by showing cost data only.

The chief of service must present to the individual, in private, the following three kinds of information:

1. "Harry, we are not talking about you personally. We are talking about three pieces of paper." (Put the discussion on an objective basis.)

2. "The first piece of paper shows that you are spending $29,000 more per month on your patients than the other members of the department. This is not the total picture, but it is just the first piece of paper."

3. "The second piece of paper is 'patient mix data' which shows that you treat about the same kind of patients as the rest of us. What this means, Harry, is that there is no need for you to tell us 'Well of course I spend more money. My patients are sicker. If you receive the tough referrals like I do, you would spend more on those patients, too.' Do you understand, Harry? We can skip that because the two pieces of paper so far indicate that you spend more money on about the same patient mix."

4. "Finally, we know that you will be concerned that we have not gone over to the other side and become so interested in the economics of health care that we have given up our professional guardianship of quality care and results for the patient. That's why we have this

third piece of paper that indicates that your complication rates and other patient results are just about like those of the rest of us."

5. *Summary*. "Harry, the point is this. The three pieces of paper show that you are spending more money than the rest of us on about the same type of patient and that your patients are not getting any weller."

6. "Harry, what do you think we should do about that?"

This sort of open, up-front approach in attempting to deal with problems and issues within the medical staff is much more likely to generate a reasonable response than the old legalistic approach of the 1970s of just "pulling the bylaws" on an individual, and having the individual surprised by a note in the mailbox that insists that he or she either do better or pack up and get out of town!

Of course, even this approach will not work with truly unreasonable, recalcitrant, unresponsive individuals. For that reason, the traditional effective adversary portions of medical staff and hospital bylaws must remain in place.

The point here is that the individual has been given an opportunity to consider objective information presented by a respected peer who holds a position of authority in the medical staff's self-governance organization.

> Only when the scenario described above takes place will any medical staff have any right to complain that administration, executives, board, and hospital managers are unduly interfering with medical staff affairs.

Figure 16-2

MEDICAL STAFF FUNCTIONS
The Old Way

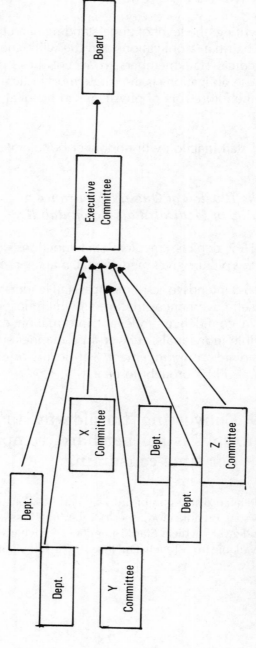

- Emphasis on Structure — Meetings & Minutes
- Arbitrary Committee Assignments — For *Everybody*
- "Cyclic Referral Syndrome" — Little Tracking of Issues from Origin to Resolution
- Little Systematic Intra-Medical Staff Communication
- Minimal Individual Responsibility

A Final Word: Fact of Life

At this writing, the level of understanding of a clinical service chief's/chairman's obligations and the willingness of responsible medical staff members to accept these positions and fulfill these obligations is the single most critical factor determining the future role of physicians in hospital leadership.[1]

Because . . .

Medical staff inaction will no longer be tolerated as an endpoint.

From the Illusion of Quality Assurance to the Reality of Medical Staff Accountability

Figure 16-2 depicts "medical staff functions" the old way. Little in this picture gives medical staff managers confidence.

Figure 16-3 intends to assist medical staff leaders with visualizing the self-governance structure in which hospital managers *can* have confidence—relevant information considered by responsible individuals, relayed in a manner suggesting that either individual improvement will occur, or organizational pressures will be brought to bear.

> Converting "the old way" to "the new way" is neither hard, complicated, nor time-consuming.

[1]For a detailed discussion of the why and how of streamlining the medical staff organization, see "More With Less—A Productive Guide to Fewer Medical Staff Committees," Richard E. Thompson, M.D., available from Teach 'Em, Inc., 160 E. Illinois Street, Chicago, IL 60611.

What is hard is accepting the new reality—genuine accountability, professionalism, and self-evaluation *are* the most protective, self-serving responses to amazing new pressures on practitioners and healthcare managers.

Figure 16-3

MEDICAL STAFF FUNCTIONS
The New Way

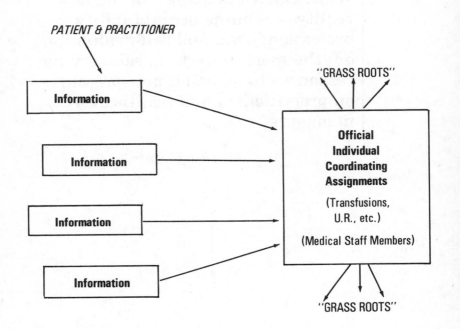

DIRECTION:
- Medical Executive Committee
- Departments
- Quality Coordinating Council

COLLECTION & DISPLAY
- QA Coordinator
- Medical Records
- Medical Staff Coordinator
- Data Processing
- Departments (e.g., Lab, X-Ray)
- Special Activities
  (e.g., Infection Control, UR, RM)

RELEVANT CLINICAL SPECIALIST(S)
- Interpretation
- Clarification
- Expand Information Base, PRN
- Education

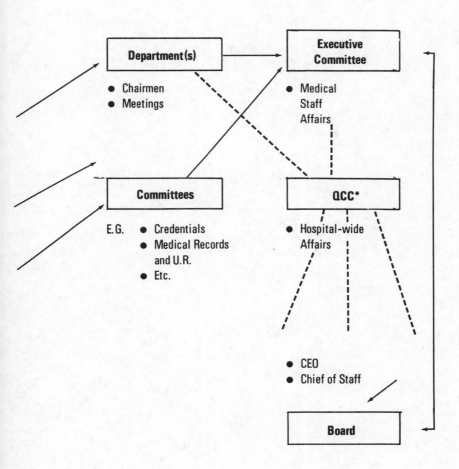

*Quality Coordinating Council

CHAPTER 17

Communication: key to success

Many who have read this book did not need to be encouraged to communicate. These individuals have always known the value of communication. On the other hand, there is nothing automatic about effective communication, and suggestions about a few specific skills may help.

Put Away Your Copy of Machiavelli

For some reason, in recent years medical staff managers may have been taught that the best way to deal with the medical staff is as circuitously and as little as possible. Not true—responsible medical staff leaders are ready for responsible institutional managers to lead them in learning effective organizational methods.

Some physicians are frightened of the times; most are not. Many would welcome upfront answers to questions that deserve answers. In the process, the institutional manager may find his or her position solidified because of increased respect and support by the now-trusting medical staff member.

Functional Communication is Better Than Structural Communication

It's easy to hide behind formally appointed groups, agendas, confidentiality, policies, minutes, and other trappings of organizational management. The best communication occurs one-to-one, often over a cup of coffee. Never assume that this is time wasted because you are only imparting information to one individual. Think about a line of cars at a stoplight. When the light changes, all the cars don't start at once. The first car starts, then the next car, then the next car, etc. One-on-one coffee-cup conversations that produce clarification, understanding, and support are productive discussions indeed.

Get Down to Brass Tacks

Neither medical staff leaders nor institutional managers should invite each other to lunch for the purpose of getting down to the nitty gritty and resolving a conflict and then spend the time discussing sports and the weather. Sometimes effective communication means taking the risk of threatening a close relationship. But when communication is carefully sought, the result is usually a strengthening and bonding between two or more individuals who can then become a nucleus for progress and success.

Use Outside Resources If You Need Them

I've traveled the country explaining DRG-payment systems to medical staffs. I can't do it any better—I can't do it as well—as many of the internal consultants available at the hospital, such as the CFO, CEO, and chief of the medical staff. My value is my objectivity—looking in from the outside. Individuals need not suspect that I will slant information I'm presenting for personal gain.

Objective communication may begin with a mutually trusted outside

resource presenting basic facts for
consideration.

A Retreat May Be the Best Way to Advance

Monthly business meetings, such as the board, medical staff
executive committee, or Joint Conference Committee, are usually planned to make it through specific agenda items as
rapidly as possible. A more relaxed retreat setting allows:

- Discovering more about ourselves, our own fears, each
  other, and each other's fears.

- A more relaxed environment that is the key to converting
  an adversary position-taking approach, to an information-sharing, problem-solving approach.

- That in separate groups, we have been saying nasty
  things about each other. Nothing softens language and
  helps us be more careful in articulating our concerns
  than being forced to modify emotions and language by
  talking in front of one another.

- Discovering that meetings can be held and views can
  be exchanged without being extremely guarded in what
  we say. At retreats, no votes need be taken. Information
  shared will be used later in traditional business meetings.
  Thus, at the retreat, individuals need not feel restrained
  and guarded in expressing their point of view, nor obli-
  gated to convert all others at this meeting to that point
  of view.

- Retreat settings thus provide an opportunity for often
  surprising and clarifying occurrences. *Example:* At a joint
  medical staff/board retreat in the textile belt of the south-

139

eastern United States, little progress had been made over several months in overcoming an impasse between the business-oriented board leaders (mostly leaders in the textile industry) and the clinically oriented medical staff members.

Within two weeks after this retreat, the impasse was resolved. It was the opinion of all present at the retreat the progress began being made when three physicians suddenly told three textile manufacturers: "Bill, Harry and John, you just can't treat patients like you make and sell socks!"

Don't Expect Automatic Harmony

A bottom line: there is absolutely no way that hospital executives, administration, managers, board members and physicians will establish any sort of effective communication if they insist on taking personally the inevitability of change in the world, and if they insist on blaming each other for it.

Pursuing the Value of Communication

Example 1: Figure 17-1 is an actual summary of the results of a joint treat. Suffice it to say that working through this brief problem list over the next few weeks and months solidified and focused joint efforts of institutional managers and medical staff leaders to deal with a variety of sticky, local problems.

Figure 17-1

"NEXT STEPS" TO CONSIDER IN FOLLOWING UP ISSUES AND CONCERNS ADDRESSED AT GOVERNING BODY/MEDICAL STAFF/ADMINISTRATION RETREAT

1. Re-examine the function and action of the Joint Conference Committee, considering the revelation in this discussion that some members of the medical staff feel that the board is not accessible enough to their needs and concerns.

2. Define "loyalty and utilization" (a) from the physician's view and (b) from the board members' view. (This and the matter of reviewing and revising the physician-selection process suggest careful, functional analysis of present medical staff bylaws.)

3. Improve systematic communication mechanisms *within* the medical staff, whether this means availability of medical staff executive committee minutes, a medical staff newsletter, use of a standardized agenda in medical staff department meetings with the department chairman charged with conveying needed information, some combination of the above, and/or other mechanisms.

4. Clarify and communicate the role and responsibilities of medical staff department chairmen, provide needed assistance with how to fulfill these responsibilities, and hold department chiefs accountable.

5. Clarify, in writing the description of objectives, functions, and "charge" of existing committees. (Specific example: Can the patient care committee be the mechanism by which nursing issues are addressed in a forum that includes at least nurses, physicians, and administration.)

6. Establish a specific protocol/procedure for flow of information when an "incident" is "investigated" — be sure the procedure includes information to (a) the medical staff, and (b) individuals involved.

7. Review the physician-selection procedure and revise/update as necessary.

8. "Take the initiative" in suggesting that 2 or 3 individuals from this hospital and St. Elsewhere "start at Square 1" to re-explore possible joint ventures and collaborative efforts, including the question of shared laboratory services. (NOTE: This was considered a dead issue because of previous impasse between the two hospitals. Discussion at the joint retreat revealed that both hospitals were now interested in pursuing this mutually beneficial venture.)

9. The board may wish to pursue the consideration of ways in which "the public" can be educated so that expectations of hospital care are reasonable.

10. The medical staff and board may wish to pursue the question of obtaining more information and/or specific assistance in dealing with a "problem practitioner," whether the problem is one of clinical judgment and practice or disruptive behavior.

Using Communication

Example 2: At a joint retreat, try the following procedure:

Step 1:   Administration, medical staff, and governing body members divide into three discussion groups.

Step 2:   Each of these three groups identifies *three* issues they consider most pressing to the hospital.

Step 3:   The administrative group keeps the issue with which it wishes to deal, gives the medical staff group an issue of concern to administration but under control of the medical staff, and presents the governing body with an issue which administration wishes the governing body would discuss.

The medical staff group keeps an issue of its own, gives one to administration, and one to the board.

The governing body group keeps an issue of its own, gives one to the medical staff, and one to administration.

Step 4:   Each group now has three issues—one issue of its own choosing, and one presented by each of the other two groups.

Step 5:   Each discussion group (still *separate* administrative, medical staff, and governing body discussion groups) now arbitrarily selects what they consider to be the most pressing of these three issues. Discussion continues.

Step 6:   After 20–30 minutes, play "musical chairs." Be sure that each of the three new discussion groups contains representatives of administration, the medical staff, and the governing body.

Step 7:   In these combined groups, continue the discussion of the most pressing issues.

Step 8:   Reconvene the group for a general discussion. Have a moderator or facilitator record the results of the discussion on a format, such as figures 17-2, 17-3, and 17-4.

Usual Results:

- A surprising clarification of concerns of each of the three groups. This occurs in spite of day-to-day contact between the same individuals thrown together in this type of special communication setting.

- Often, a surprising agreement on what the one or two central major issues in the hospital are.

- Often, a new, balanced appreciation of concerns, fears and blocks to resolving the key issues.

- Finally, of course (imperative), a list of no more than eight or ten next steps to be taken by administration, the medical staff, the governing body, and/or combined groups in *finally* achieving mutually beneficial and productive joint efforts in resolving critical issues.

(NOTE: This type of retreat can be conducted with an outside facilitator or consultant. It may also be discovered that within representatives of administration, the medical staff, and governing body are individuals with the skills to lead this kind of productive discussion.)

The "Is This A Good Decision" Checklist

Example 3: One of the most counterproductive and disruptive habits we have developed in the last few years is to jump on bandwagons—to reach for an off-the-shelf, *quick fix* solution without considering both the immediate and long-range consequences of our actions.

Figure 17-2

MEDICAL STAFF

SOURCE	THE ISSUE	NEXT STEPS
KEPT		
FROM GOVERNING BODY		
FROM ADMINISTRATION		

Figure 17-3

ADMINISTRATION

SOURCE	THE ISSUE	NEXT STEPS
KEPT		
FROM MEDICAL STAFF		
FROM GOVERNING BODY		

Figure 17-4

GOVERNING BODY

SOURCE	THE ISSUE	NEXT STEPS
KEPT		
FROM MEDICAL STAFF		
FROM ADMINISTRATION		

Before deciding on any action plan, medical staff managers and medical staff leaders might avoid serious consequences by applying this checklist (figure 17-5) to their decision before proceeding with it.

Again, while these suggestions about communication may seem to be talking down to experienced managers and medical staff leaders, their use is only suggested because they have served many times to be the keys to resolving what were previously considered absolute impasses.

Using Communication

Example 4: A short, monthly version of the joint retreat: The No Surprises/Nice Surprises Council.

An increasing number of hospitals are finding one to two hours a month for an unofficial, informal meeting between interested representatives of administration, the board, and medical staff members who wish to come. The agenda of this meeting consists of each group sharing only two major issues of current concern. No votes are taken, but resulting discussions and actions are reflected in official meetings of official authority groups.

For the meeting to be successful, it starts on time and ends an hour and fifteen minutes later, without respect to getting through a certain agenda. No existing formal or legal structure in hospital or corporate bylaws, including the Joint Conference Committee, matches this communicative function since these more formal groups follow procedures designed to deal with specific crises and problems.

Figure 17-6 is a sample of the results of one meeting of such a "No Surprises/Nice Surprises" Council.

Figure 17-5

SUGGEST: BOLD STEP — ● *Before* final decision
                        ● *Before* feasibility study

Make yourselves discuss:

Why do we want to do this ???
(Restructure, merge, have a teaching program, go on a retreat)

Plus your list

☐ Revenue

☐ Patient/Community Service-Convenience

☐ PR/Image

☐ Ethics

☐ Medical Staff Service/Convenience

☐ "Marketing" Value

☐ Crowd Out "The Competition"

☐ Enhance the Teaching Program

☐ Ego — "We're the cat's meow!"

☐ Attract New Physicians (of certain kinds)?

☐ Do our part to relieve the fear — panic many people feel about high cost of health care ("some scary day")

☐ Change public image from reactionary to pro-active (capture the initiative)

☐ Short-range Benefit

☐ Long-range Benefit

☐ Basically, because it appears to be the fashionable thing to do right now.

☐ Other

☐ Other

☐ Other

**Anticipated Impact on Medical Staff
Trust/Participation/Support**

    ☐ None

    ☐ Positive

    ☐ Oops!

If "Oops!" — Why???

    ☐ Decision/implementation is substantive threat to (a) medical staff organization, or (b) significant number of individual staff appointees.

    ☐ Lack of understanding for need to do this at this time. ("Unnecessary," "top-heavy management")

    ☐ Unhappy (furious!) with *way* the decision was made ("surprise!").

    ☐ Effective Dr. Trouble ("George doesn't like anything...")

    ☐ "This problem starts 30 years ago..."

Additional steps and/or modifications in decision as a result of applying these two checklists: _____

_____

_____

_____

_____

Figure 17-6

**LIST OF ISSUES DISCUSSED AT THE APRIL "NO SURPRISES" COUNCIL,
WITH A LISTING OF EXPECTATIONS FOR FOLLOW-UP**

1. Criteria for deciding an overall bed allocation will be presented for discussion at next month's meeting of the "No Surprises" Council. These will *not* be absolute numbers, but a listing of factors upon which the allocation numbers will be based.

   The present goal for having numerical allocation decided on and announced is one month after completion of construction of the new building.

   Representatives of the medical staff indicated that this listing would certainly be progress in relieving concern about plans for the future of (xxxxx) Hospital.

2. There will be a special meeting of the Quality Assurance Committee about a problem of marginal practice, raised at this meeting by representatives of the medical staff.

3. The medical staff might be able to help with the dollar problems of the board caused by Medicaid cutbacks. This will be placed on the agenda of the Medical Executive Committee.

4. The reasons for and procedure used on "administrative rounds" will be explained to the medical staff since there apparently are rumors that "administration is checking on the doctors' orders."

5. At the suggestions of medical staff representatives, Mr. Mixler, current chairman of the hospital board, will serve as the monthly moderator of the No Surprises/Nice Surprises Council sessions.

You've got to believe it—*mis*understanding is the norm.

Avoidance of misunderstanding—avoidance of arguing when we do not really disagree—avoidance of seeing sinister motives where none exist—require new management buzzwords—information sharing, cooperative effort, careful selection of language and definitions, and numerous opportunities to "get together," if for no other reason than to dispel suspicion and innuendo produced (and often depended upon) by small splinter groups.

CHAPTER 18

A summary—
errors to avoid

There is no need for anyone, regardless of his or her skills or background, to believe that the complex economic, ethical, legal, and image problems of the health-care industry can be addressed in splendid isolation. The CFO who asks, "How can *I* handle economic malpractice?" is making the mistake of attempting to deal with issues in splendid isolation. But, so is the practitioner who continues to cling to now-obsolete clichés such as, "The government's not going to tell me how to practice medicine," "Only doctors understand patient care," and "This whole thing is the fault of the politicians and investigative reporters."

It's hard to avoid the tunnel-vision, me-only, counterproductive attitude, especially since we became so conditioned to a disjointed, "me-only" society in the 1970s.

An example of this tunnel-vision: While audio-visual aids were set up at the beginning of one hospital's weekend retreat, the hotel banquet manager in charge of refreshments and arrangements appeared in the room. She was asked, "Could we have our coffee now?" Her reply was, "Sure. Are you the Danish group?" The preoccupied reply was, "No. We're from Port Washington, Indiana."

All the manager wanted to know was if we wanted sweet rolls with the coffee. Those who were preparing for the meeting were concerned only with their own identity and problems.

> Believe it: The new realities require balanced skills and priorities between those who understand healthcare as big business, and those who understand it as compassionate caring.

Learn to Avoid Argumentative Traps Into Which People Expect Us to Fall

Physicians "licensed to practice medicine and surgery in all its branches" continued to argue that this distinguishes them from "limited practitioners." The new reality is that the complexities of patient care make *everyone* a limited practitioner in one way or another.

Similarly, managers conditioned to think that structure is an endpoint may continue to trap themselves by responding to what financial and legal advisors tell them is important, without heeding the practical, functional realities of a hospital— the things their professional staff tells them are important.

Don't Argue That Money Can Only Be Saved in Healthcare by Impairing Quality

Nobody believes that anymore. It simply is not true. Having had a recent hospital experience, it was discouraging to be reminded that once an individual becomes a hospitalized patient, he or she becomes viewed in a certain way. An individual recovering from surgery at home would eat three meals a day, perform normal bodily functions, and go about the activities of daily living. But, as long as the recuperating patient is in the hospital, it seems absolutely imperative to those caring for the patient that "vital signs" be taken and recorded (usually following an established protocol that has little to do with the specific medical problem of the patient), and that serum electrolytes be drawn, duly posted on the chart, and reviewed daily.

In healthcare, both institutional managers and practitioners do a lot through force of habit, rather than through proven, tested impact on patient-care results.

> Even when it comes to rationing healthcare, don't fall into the trap of arguing that the American health-care system has never previously made decisions about who obtains the benefits of complex, costly medical procedures.

Never Assume That Economic, Legal, and Ethical Issues Are Separate Questions

Especially in health care, it is impossible to make an economic decision without considering its impact on individuals. Conversely, it is equally impossible for practitioners to make individual clinical decisions anymore without considering the economics of health care.

Don't Be Disqualified From Controlling Your Own Destiny

The new realities of health care are so distasteful to some that they will:

- withdraw from the arena.

- continue to believe that adversary, combative approaches are more productive in the long run than mutual cooperative problem-solving efforts.

Consider the Hospital as a Whole

The "3-legged" stool—administration, the board, and medical staff—has done little in recent years to approach issues in nursing. It is encouraging at this writing that a national organization such as the American Hospital Association and an accreditation agency such as the JCAH are beginning to sound as if reasonable voices respectfully raised can be heeded to the mutual benefit of all concerned.

Never Fail to Pay Attention to "Base Business"

In addition to jumping on the bandwagon of recruiting new physicians to a community in an activity considered self-protective, perhaps there will be a restoration of genuine concern with suggestions and interests of committed practitioners already on the hospital staff.

In addition, the successful hospital managers and practitioners will be those who forego superficiality and artificiality in marketing. A short time ago, the Hertz car rental company advertised that they beat the competition three ways:

- When you rent a little, you get nice gifts.

- When you rent a lot, you get nice gifts.

- Whether you rent a little or a lot, you get both free gifts and travel.

The disturbing point was the absence of attention to base business in this marketing approach. Where is the component of the ad that says the car one rents will run?

> **Neither hospital managers nor practitioners can afford to go overboard in the direction of marketing and business incentives without paying equal attention to their professional heritage and mission.**

CHAPTER 19

Where do we go from here?

Brainstorm

A combined group of medical staff, administration and board leaders should now meet for the purpose of brainstorming. Use some of the new approaches and assumptions suggested here. Consider:

- *Modification*—even radical modification—of present activities and decisions. This is not done for the sake of being radical, but because new, major successes now require new, major initiatives.

- *A re-ordering of priorities.* Should decisions about exact formats of new economic joint ventures be tabled until basic joint understanding between managers and practitioners has been achieved?

- *Are you really starting at square 1?* Or do sophisticated hospital managers possess understanding that practitioners with clinical backgrounds do not? If that is true, would it not be unwise to skip the step of expanding the basis of support for needed initiatives?

- *Are you being upfront?* Manipulative management styles have not produced buzzwords associated with security and success in the healthcare field.

- *Has enough front-end time been spent considering and agreeing upon both short-range objectives and long-range goals?* Have parameters that can be used to measure progress toward these goals and objectives been adequately established?

- *Have you carefully selected methods of approach that are related to your stated goals and objectives?* Don't fool yourself. Don't pick a method because it appears to be the safest way to go.

- *Have you stopped looking for quick fixes?*

- *Have you taken yourself out of the fix the blame mode and put yourself into the fix the problem mode?*

- *Have you stopped being a uni-dimensional thinker?* There's never been a problem that didn't have more than one cause.

- *Are you responsive to change?* If you want things to stay at all the same, you may have to accept some changes.

- *Have you considered effective use of the successful hospital manager's/practitioner's secret weapon:* genuine accountability for decisions which produce productivity in the healthcare field.

- *Have you thought about "the bottomline?"* If all else fails . . .

> Pretend you're the patient. We are all likely to need the services of the healthcare system some day. If you practice the procedures examined in this book, patients, administrators, board members, and medical staff will benefit.